# SACRED PLANT
# INITIATIONS

"The world is in crisis because modern societies have bought into a story of separateness. Plants have taught cultures throughout the ages a story of interconnectedness. This beautiful, magical, wonderful book is a re-initiation into teachings that we are a part of—not apart from—nature, teachings from the plants themselves that are essential for the very survival of our species. Carole Guyett is a modern shaman, an inspiration!"

JOHN PERKINS, AUTHOR OF
*CONFESSIONS OF AN ECONOMIC HIT MAN, SHAPESHIFTING,*
AND *THE WORLD IS AS YOU DREAM IT*

"Carole's clear instructions, along with her loving encouragement for personal creative additions, are designed to guide the readers into how to have their own uniquely valuable, magical, and practical plant experiences. Plants are indeed our elders and teachers, and this book will help any sincere seeker to reawaken to their own true nature, and that is the most healing gift of all."

ROBIN ROSE BENNETT, HERBALIST AND AUTHOR OF
*THE GIFT OF HEALING HERBS* AND *HEALING MAGIC*

"An extraordinary, inspirational, and highly practical guide to exploring the spiritual realms of plants and opening gateways to healing and transformation. Carole gives a whole new meaning to 'plant diets' and beautifully describes how journeying into the inner world of plants gives you a sense of oneness with everything in creation. This is the perfect book for anyone wishing to deepen their connection to the plant world."

ANNE MCINTYRE, MEDICAL HERBALIST, AYURVEDIC
PRACTITIONER, AND AUTHOR OF *THE AYURVEDA BIBLE*

"Bravo! *Sacred Plant Initiations* gives readers a unique perspective in working with plants and discovering their generous gifts. The plant dieting ceremonies Carole describes are inspiring, informative, and provide a clear lens into an original and sacred means of communion with nature. The knowledge shared in this book is vast and indispensable to anyone studying plants or seeking healing and transformation."

NICKI SCULLY, AUTHOR OF *POWER ANIMAL MEDITATIONS*, *ALCHEMICAL HEALING*, AND *PLANETARY HEALING*

"Groundbreaking, inspiring, and destined to become a classic. Carole Guyett's approach is grounded, original, and practical. She takes the reader deep into an understanding of the spiritual character of plants and their associated spirits. *Sacred Plant Initiations* is an important step forward in healing our relationship with nature and restoring balance to our beautiful planet. A beautiful book."

WILLIAM BLOOM, PH.D., AUTHOR OF *THE POWER OF THE NEW SPIRITUALITY* AND *WORKING WITH ANGELS*

"I would recommend this book to anyone who is interested in cross-communication between humans and other species. The simplicity and the wisdom speak for themselves as does the inherent charm in Carole's style."

JUDITH HOAD, HERBALIST, VIBRATIONAL MEDICINE PRACTITIONER, AND AUTHOR OF *HEALING WITH HERBS*

"A beautifully written book, full of deep insights and concrete and practical instructions to become a modern-times plant alchemist. As you read it, you'll feel the doors of a magical world open, a world of interconnectedness, healing, and joy that we all remember and long for. Carole's expertise and love guide us to recognize that plants are a part of us, and when we relate to them with reverence we reawaken parts of our soul, realizing that this is, indeed, what they truly are."

ESPERIDE ANANAS, HEALER AND AUTHOR OF *MUSIC OF THE PLANTS*

# SACRED PLANT INITIATIONS

## Communicating with Plants for
## Healing and Higher Consciousness

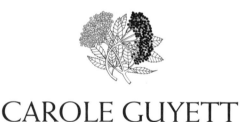

## CAROLE GUYETT

Bear & Company
Rochester, Vermont • Toronto, Canada

Bear & Company
One Park Street
Rochester, Vermont 05767
www.BearandCompanyBooks.com

Bear & Company is a division of Inner Traditions International

**Library of Congress Cataloging-in-Publication Data**
Guyett, Carole.
  Sacred plant initiations : communicating with plants for healing and higher
consciousness / Carole Guyett.
      pages cm
  Includes bibliographical references and index.
  ISBN 978-1-59143-213-5 (pbk.) — ISBN 978-1-59143-214-2 (e-book)
  1. Plants—Miscellanea. 2. Rites and ceremonies. I. Title.
  BF1623.P5G89 2015
  133'.258—dc23
                                                                    2014031980

Printed and bound in the United States by McNaughton & Gunn, Inc.

10  9  8  7  6  5  4  3  2  1

Text design and layout by Priscilla Baker
This book was typeset in Garamond Premier Pro with Shelley Script, Weiss,
Adobe Jenson Pro, and Gill Sans used as display typefaces
Illustrations by Judith Evans

To send correspondence to the author of this book, mail a first-class letter to the
author c/o Inner Traditions • Bear & Company, One Park Street, Rochester, VT
05767, and we will forward the communication, or contact the author directly
through her website at **www.derrynagittah.ie**.

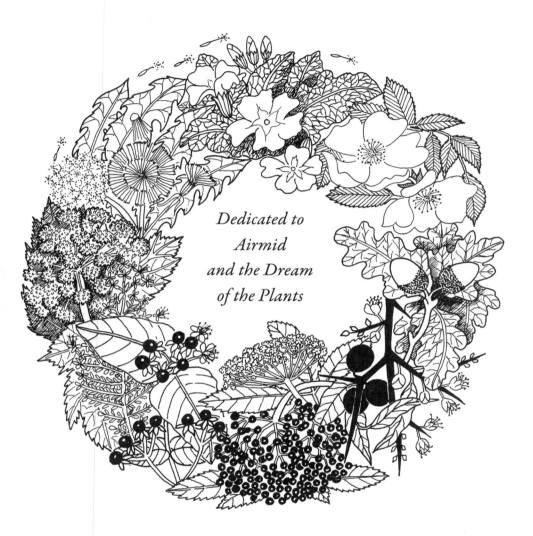

*Dedicated to*
*Airmid*
*and the Dream*
*of the Plants*

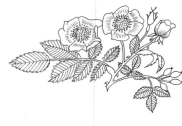

# Contents

PART 2

# ENTERING THE DREAM
# OF THE PLANTS
*Sacred Plant Initiations for the
Eight Fire Festivals*

# Becoming Truly Human

*M*y first plant initiation began in the spring of 2010 while I was in rural England on a work assignment teaching GreenBreath and plant communication to a group of interested students. The plan was for a relatively simple and consolidated round trip, including time on the front end to touch down in Ireland for a few precious days with my so distant yet close friend Carole Guyett. Days later in the course of teaching in England, I happened early one morning to take notice of a vast array of little yellow Primroses painting the hillside behind my lovely little guest cottage in the Cornwall countryside. I had never seen so many in one place, certainly not at home in Vermont where *Primulus vulgaris* ordinarily lives as a cultivated plant instead of one wildly covering hillsides.

The time passed well. However, when winding up the class and departing for London for my return the next day to the States, all civilized plans began to turn to dust (or ash as the case may be) for the news on the wind was that a powerful volcanic eruption was occurring in Iceland and spewing tremendous ash clouds into the air. Due to shifting air currents over land and sea, airlines were becoming powerless to fly as scheduled. On any given day whole airports were shut down so that European and international travel came to a halt.

I had only one night booked in London and once I found that I would not be flying home the next morning, I went into a mild panic wondering where I would stay. Thousands of people were in the same predicament trying to go somewhere but unable to. After many hours of tearful communications back home with my husband, Mark, we decided the best plan was for me to try to make my way to the coast for a boat back to Ireland where Carole and her husband Steve might provide much needed assistance and comfort for me under these circumstances. I was scared, exhausted, and worrying about getting home for my apprentice-ship course beginning five days later. If I could just get back to Ireland, I would at least be comfortable even if I was stranded in a foreign land.

All the boats sailing across the Irish Sea were booked except one middle-of-the-night boat that traveled to the southern port of Rosslare. It was the only possible way to get back to Ireland and so I decided I would try to make it. But I was in London, a country girl in a city of eight million people trying to negotiate getting to a boat to take me to Ireland with no cell phone, map, or helping hand. I inquired at the hotel desk how to get to the train that would take me to the boat that would take me to Ireland. She calmly pointed out the door and said, "Stand on that corner and wait for the red bus." Do you know how many red buses there are in London going to innumerable different locations? As I stood there watching one red bus after another go by with my two suitcases, backpack, and large frame drum hanging off my shoulder, a large tear found its way down my cheek. I knew it was time to make a shift, and as my friend Rocio would say, to begin to "manage the forces." I thought of all those little Primroses on that English hillside and a smile came to my face, a deep breath fol-lowed, and I gathered myself to ask for help.

My initiation had begun.

I stood at the bus stop and called on my "tower of strength" ally, White Pine. "I need help here; I really can't do this alone." Suddenly an angel appeared in the form of an English businessman of Indian ancestry. He asked me where I was going and I said Ireland. He proceeded to tell me this bus, that train, then another train, get off here, go there, and then find the ferry. I looked at him with what must have been a shocked wide-eyed stare, at which point he said, "I'll take you to the train." As I stood, com-pletely at his mercy, I heard the words of my mother, "Don't ever go off with a stranger." I gave him a quick scan and checked in with my heart—it went "ping." I got on the bus with him and off we went. He safely delivered me to the train after the bus ride and helped me buy the correct ticket to the boat that would deliver me to Ireland. He walked to the platform with me to make sure I was on the right train and then said, "Goodbye and good luck." "Wait," I said, "please, what is your name?" "Hans," he replied and I said, "Thank you, and my name is Pam." He turned and was gone. I got on the train and sat in a daze wondering who he *really* was—a British-accented Indian named Hans—wow!

After three trains and an all-night ferry across the Irish Sea, I arrived in Ireland at 6:15 a.m. to find Carole's husband Steve waiting for me on the dock (after a three-hour drive from his home in Clare) saying, "Can I take your bags, mate?" I fell into his arms in a heap with the most gratitude I had experienced in a long time.

Once back at Carole's home, she immersed me in preparations for a Primrose initiation she was offering for Bealtaine (or Beltane) on May 1. We roamed the lanes and countryside picking beautiful little flowers with heart-shaped petals to make into an infusion for the plant elixir. I had the great fortune of helping Carole every step of the way and when it came time to make the elixir, I also was privy to her very conscious intentions to prepare the dieting mixture in a ceremonial way. I felt I was being given a great gift by being at the right hand of a high priestess. After making the preparation she gave me a bottle of it to bring home so I could have my own ritual at the same time she and her group were doing their diet in Ireland.

So much happened during my solitary Primrose diet! I knew I needed to rededicate my life to the plants, deeper than I had ever gone before. It was time to fearlessly walk into the unknown, trusting that my power is my love—my love for the Earth and all her beings, especially the plants and the trees. Just as I began my initiation in an unknown circumstance— with an unknown person in an unknown place and an unknown timing for when I would be home—I trusted my plant allies to help me and they did. Primrose is known as the Key Flower and she surely gave me the key to my greatest strength.

When I look back on this experience, I realize that if there hadn't been a volcanic eruption while I happened to be in England, I would never have had the opportunity to be with Carole while she prepared for the Primrose initiation and I wouldn't have done the initiation myself. I stepped into the dreamtime of Primrose before the volcano erupted, and as I wrote in my journal, "I'm walking in a spiral with a clear quartz stone at the center. The quartz is like a beaming station—beaming me, with the help of Primrose, to my White Pine tree at home. My energy body is preparing to travel home, physically home, but more so, home to myself." Later I wrote, "These plants are asking us to investigate the questions, 'Who am I and what am I doing here?' They are pushing us to be who we truly are, to be truly human." This was a profoundly deep experience of a plant urging me to step fully into my inherent creative power of being human, and realize that, as Carole says, "The plants can help us to develop as mature human beings and truly walk this Earth as sacred humans."

In traditional initiatory cultures such as the Dagara tribe of West Africa, the highland Maya of Guatemala, and the aborigines of Australia, there is an understanding that to be initiated means to cross a further threshold into one's maturity in order to take up a place of responsibility and belonging within the community. The community as a whole serves as the container that holds within it all the vitality of the village. An initiate pushes edges by confronting demons and deities who flirt with death. Through a ritual journey of dismemberment, the initiate dies to be born anew. As one is born anew into the wholeness of his or her being, a deep understanding arises that initiation is not about becoming a better person necessarily, but more about being in fuller, more realized relationship with Spirit. By feeding the Divine through ceremony, all of life is fed and the community thrives. Modernity has distorted the natural initiatory setting, relegating it merely to such forms as college fraternities, military encampments, or corporate board rooms. This poor imitation of a true initiation rings hollow in the face of a community container that holds initiates in its embrace. And yet, how are we modern, civilized people to be initiated in an authentic way, a way that serves the whole ecology—the human and the more than human? And what of the elders, and where have they all gone? Without them, who will initiate us?

What Carole Guyett is bringing to the world is a new form of initiation. She invites us to seek those we are most closely related to—plants—to become our initiators. Carole has formed a community of plant dreamers, holding the container within which to carry out the ceremony of initiation once again. Now our elders, the plants, are initiating us into being true humans who take up our rightful place of belonging in the wider world of Nature.

Now that I have participated in, and guided, several plant initiations, I have come to know that not only psychotropic plants but *all* plants are "Teacher Plants." There is so much to learn from each and every plant. When treated with honor, respect, and loving kindness in co-creative partnership, all plants and trees respond accordingly. In plant initiations the plants are worked with in sacred ceremony every step of the way— from the very first time one begins to gather the plants, to the making of and ingesting of the elixir, to dreaming with the plant, to the hands-on experience with the plant, and beyond. When the plants are treated in this fashion their teachings and guidance are limitless. I have come to recognize that the familiar Buddhist saying rings true with plants: "When the student is ready the teacher appears." For I see that when people are ready plants offer them one more piece to aid in their growth. For myself, I have learned from plants through sensory awareness, felt sensation, light, song, and quite unexpectedly, by way of a volcanic eruption leading to an initiation. The plants and trees are clearly available to us at this critical juncture in our journey. They guide us in knowing that the Earth is our home and plants are our kin, that we do remember their language, and we can take up our rightful place in the vast web of Nature that gives us our very life.

As I read through *Sacred Plant Initiations* I am inspired time and time again as I am drawn into the full being-ness of each plant. It is not just one aspect of the plant I am being invited to get to know but instead the wholeness of the plant. As one initiate shares, "Each plant is a book." I find myself loving the deepening of my relations with old friends, as when a best friend tells you something personal you never knew before or a piece you had forgotten and now are so happy to rediscover. I also experience much joy in getting to know someone new like Blackthorn, who turns out to be "sloe." Throughout this wonderful book I find a bright light is shed on an aspect of my dear friend Carole, which in the past I had only glimpsed but now see so clearly—Carole walks her talk and is deeply dedicated to the plants. It makes me weep with gratitude to know there are people such as this fine woman walking the planet right now. Carole is a dreamer who walks in simultaneous worlds of the seen and the unseen. She acknowledges the interconnection that goes on between the worlds and weaves her own magic into the exquisite tapestry of walking with Spirit on a daily basis. There's none other who can bring you these teachings with such genuine authority and with such an unassuming heart of gold.

The book you hold in your hands is one whose time has come. The plants and trees are calling us to take up our rightful place and reclaim our birthright of being a part of Nature, not separate from it. They are asking us to remember who we are, where we live, and how to live. They are guiding us in our evolution to know the truth of our lineage as sacred humans, those who walk with Spirit and aliveness each and every day.

PAM MONTGOMERY

Pam Montgomery is an author, teacher, and practitioner who passionately embraces her role as a spokesperson for the green beings. She has been investigating plants and their intelligent spiritual nature for more than three decades. She is the author of two books, one of which is the highly acclaimed *Plant Spirit Healing: A Guide to Working with Plant Consciousness.* She teaches internationally about plant spirit healing and spiritual ecology, and that people are nature evolutionaries. She is a founding member of United Plant Savers and more recently of the Organization of Nature Evolutionaries, or O.N.E. Her latest research is on the light and sound of plants, which are foundational means of communication in the biological world. She lives in Vermont and, with her husband Mark, operates the Partner Earth Education Center at Sweetwater Sanctuary.

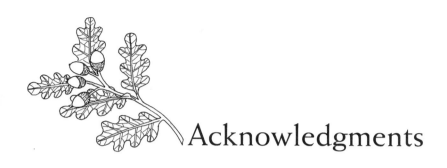

# Acknowledgments

*G*rateful thanks go to everyone who has taken part in the plant diets I have led and especially to those who have generously shared their stories. Many of your names have been changed to protect your privacy, but you know who you are, and the book would not have been possible without your valued contributions. Particular thanks go to my treasured friends and labyrinth sisters Martina, Rose, and Joan. I am forever grateful for your constant loving hearts, endless support, good humor, and practical assistance. You are angels in human form.

Thanks to Judith for your beautiful illustrations and to Rowan and Erin for your photographs. Gratitude to Henrique for your lovely flute playing, to Tommy for lending us instruments, and to Ruth for passing on the Key Flower story. Thanks also to Camaleonte from Damanhur for assisting me with the plant biofeedback device, thereby allowing us to hear the songs of the plants.

Thanks to Liz for diligently reading the manuscript and giving so much sensible advice. Gratitude to the team at Inner Traditions, especially my helpful and understanding editors, Laura Schlivek and Claire Diamond; you have been a pleasure to work with. Thanks to Penny for your advice at the start of this project and to Eleanor for holding the connection with Islay.

Grateful thanks to Arwyn, whose wise teachings have shaped my work. Blessings to you and Tree for your generous hearts, your unfailing support, and your inspiring commitment to a Dream of Beauty. I would also like to thank Dawn and my teachers, guides, and helpers from all of the worlds who have offered so much support and guidance for this book. Boundless thanks go to the plants who are always there for me. I am honored and privileged to be in your service.

Immeasurable thanks go to my dear soul sister Pam. Heartfelt gratitude for the gifts of your love and friendship, and for our shared dreams and dedication to the plant world. Our bond is a rare and precious thing, and I give thanks for your presence in my life. Your enthusiastic encouragement has driven me onward and your constant support has kept this book afloat when it might otherwise have floundered. Bless you for your generous advice, for your detailed comments on the original manuscript, and for giving me an American perspective. Further gratitude to you, Mark, for the comfort of your outstandingly warm heart.

Thanks to Carol and Yukari and to all my loving and supportive family and friends. Particular thanks go to my wonderful sons, Josh and Rory. You are bright, shining lights in my life and your influence on this book has been immense. Thanks for your laughter and love, for your inspiration and philosophical discussions, your computer skills, your cooking, and so much more. Special thanks for taking on the audio tracks and bringing such expertise, dedication, and fun to the project.

Finally, I send thanks to my beloved husband, Steve, brave and stronghearted enough to share this journey. I give thanks for your precious love and commitment and for always believing in me. Thank you for your guardianship, humor, and support and for honoring my dream. I love you.

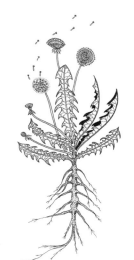

# Introduction

*Sacred and Holy Ones of the Plant World,*
*We come to you with honoring and respect,*
*We come seeking to align ourselves with your Dream,*
*To be in right relationship with you*
*And to know your ways of Beauty.*
*Beloved Ones, our hearts are open and full of gratitude.*
*May our lives be a Sacred Offering of Beauty*
*In service to the Plants and all the Worlds of*
*Grandmother Earth.*

This book is written for all those who would like to deepen their relationship with plants and Nature.* It describes methods that can transform your relationship with the plant world, with yourself, and with life itself. Described here are plant diets, sacred ceremonies that offer powerful initiations by the plant world. *Plant dieting* is a traditional term referring to a wide range of practices undertaken in order to form a profound relationship with a plant and to receive its gifts, particularly for guidance and healing. This book presents a way of experiencing

---

*Throughout this book certain words are capitalized that would not normally be so in common English usage. The reason is to sanctify and accord value to certain aspects of life. Naturally, everything in life is sacred, but my intention is to bring routine awareness to the sacredness of certain key energies.

plants as conscious spiritual beings and aims to demonstrate how common plants in our hedgerows provide a form of medicine that can help us take an evolutionary leap to a new vision of reality.

Ceremonial plant dieting is a traditional method of honoring the plant world. The ceremonial process offers a unique way to connect deeply with all aspects of a plant, opening gateways to spiritual realms and facilitating powerful transformation at physical, emotional, mental, and spiritual levels. While the knowledge and practice of ceremonial plant dieting has been largely forgotten in Western society, these traditions remain intact in many indigenous communities throughout the world. Most well-known, contemporary plant diets are associated with psychoactive plants. However, the plant ceremonies described in this book involve powerful, sacred ceremonies undertaken with nonpsychoactive, native Irish plants. As far as I am aware, this is a unique work as the experience of dieting nonpsychoactive, native Irish plants has never before been researched in this way. Many of the featured plants are widespread throughout the planet. Given that this book is being published in the United States, I have sought to show their availability in North America and elsewhere. (Readers may note that the text has been edited to bring it into alignment with American styles of spelling, punctuation, and wording.)

There are many ways of dieting with plants, including a variety of purposes, approaches, and durations. On one level, a plant diet may simply consist of the regular ingestion of a single plant in order to receive its physical benefits. The plant diets described in this book, however, are carried out within the context of sacred ceremony, explicitly acknowledging and honoring the unique spiritual and physical signatures of the plants being dieted. The plant is our sacrament and offers us communion with Spirit. By working in a sacred manner we can be the recipients of many gifts and we can also give back and be of service to the plant world. The gifts received can benefit both the individual and the collective, giving an opportunity to heal imbalances we may have created in the Web of Life.

What is shared in these pages arises from my work with plants over the last thirty years and, particularly from the past decade, my quest to develop native plant diets. In 2008 I began undertaking these diets with a group of committed people in the west of Ireland. For a number of years we carried out plant diets coinciding with our celebratory ceremonies for the seasonal Fire Festivals.* Over time, these diets were extended to the wider community and they continue to be offered to my friends, apprentices, and to the public. Material included in this book represents the documented experiences of participants, their words having been left as close as possible to verbatim, corrections only being made for clarity and American usage. Though many participants did not initially have strong connections with plants, through their participation in these ceremonies they have undergone profound changes in their relationships with the plant world and with all of life.

At this time on our planet, vast numbers of humans have become disconnected from Spirit and the natural world. This sense of separateness has led to a planetary crisis point where humans are capable of immeasurable destruction. At the same time, people have a yearning to reconnect with Nature. More and more of us are actively seeking ways to live in harmony with the planet and all of life. This book offers a way to connect with Spirit through the plant world. It is a way to develop a relationship of honor and respect for all beings. When we perceive the consciousness and spiritual quality of plants, we are much more likely to care for them as we do for ourselves, realizing that we are all equal and accountable for our actions. Likewise, when we feel our connection and perceive ourselves to be part of all of life on Earth then it becomes instinctive to care for our planet rather than to cause damage.

My hope is that through this book, readers will be touched by the wisdom and healing of the plants and may be inspired to carry out their own ceremonial plant diets. These ceremonies are easy! They are not reserved for an elite few. I aim to provide clear guidance and simple instructions that will enable you to design and experience your own plant diets in a way that is appropriate for you and the plants around you. If you love plants, it

---

*The eight main traditional pagan festivals (all referred to as Fire Festivals in this book) celebrate the turning of the Wheel of the Year and comprise the pre-Celtic festivals of Winter Solstice, Spring Equinox, Summer Solstice, and Autumn Equinox together with the Celtic Fire Festivals of Samhain, Brigid's Day, Bealtaine, and Lughnasadh.

can be sheer ecstasy to spend focused time in the intimate presence of one of your beloveds.

Life on planet Earth is at a turning point. The whole of Grandmother Earth and Her worlds are evolving. I use the term *Grandmother* because in this process of evolution the Earth Herself is moving from Mother to Grandmother. The *worlds of Grandmother Earth* refers to all realms of planet Earth—mineral, plant, animal, and human. We are all part of one organism and all of us are evolving, albeit at different rates. As humans, we need to evolve rapidly if we are to survive as a species. It is my understanding that the plant world is offering to help us evolve to a new level of consciousness including genetic change and the modification of our DNA. Plants are leading the way, offering keys to our awakening, while helping us to expand our awareness and initiating us into what it truly means to live as sacred human beings on this planet. Throughout this book, the terms *plant diet* and *plant initiation* are used interchangeably since these plant diets are initiation ceremonies that can take us to a new level. An initiation strips away our familiar beliefs and opens our consciousness to new possibilities.

It is my intention in this book to demonstrate how ceremonial plant diets provide this kind of initiation. The plant world can help each of us to live a more fulfilling, productive life in harmony with Nature as we become more fully ourselves. Ceremonial plant diets provide a safe and accessible way to receive the sacred teachings from the plants. It is my strong and heartfelt hope and desire that this book will inspire you to discover and deepen the joy of your own rich journey with the plant world. May it bring heart blessings to you and to all of life on Earth.

*BLESSED BE*

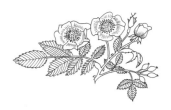

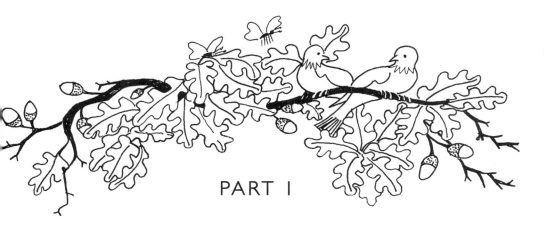

PART I

# Sacred Plant Initiations
# for Modern Times

CONNECTING with
PLANT CONSCIOUSNESS for
PERSONAL and PLANETARY
TRANSFORMATION

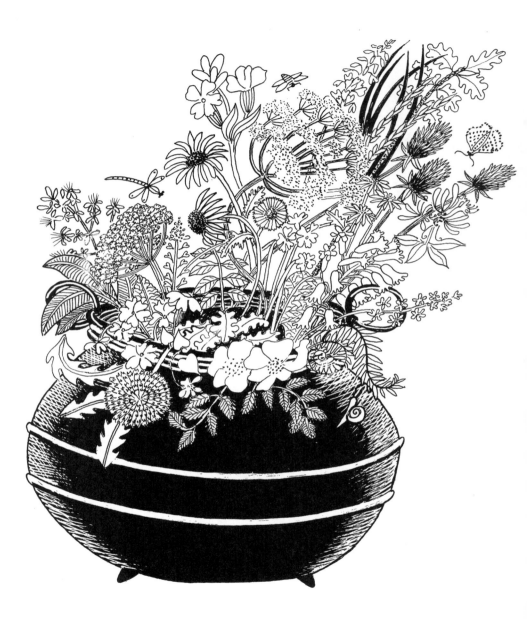

*A sacred cauldron of abundance overflowing with native plants*

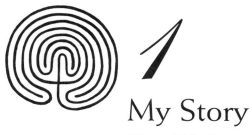

# 1
# My Story
## How We Started Dieting Plants at Derrynagittah

*Hail Ancestors of this Sacred Land*
*Place of nourishment and inspiration.*
*Hail Ancestors of blood who gave us life,*
*Womb to womb and breath to Sacred breath.*
*Hail Ancestors of Spirit, Guides, and Teachers*
*You from behind the veil who show us the Beauty of Life.*
*Ancestors we come in thanks for your innumerable gifts.*
*May you be honored*
*May you be forever blessed.*

orn and raised in England, I grew up with a deep love of plants and as a young child I lived in a world of nature spirits, fairies, and magnificent spiritual beings. You can imagine my surprise at being told that this was all in my head, or worse still, that I was making it up! I soon learned not to mention these magical encounters, and it was not long before they ceased to happen. My love of plants continued on, and some of my happiest moments were spent in Nature with the flowers and trees as my friends. As with many children, it was my great delight to make potions and lotions. I remember at age eleven making breast-enhancement creams for my less-well-endowed school friends!

It was my passionate interest in both plants and healing that led, in my twenties, to my training as a medical herbalist at the School of Herbal Medicine in England. During these same four years, I met and studied with a Wise Woman or hedgewitch* whose knowledge of traditional healing and the Old Ways (the term used for the spiritual beliefs and practices of those who follow this ancient path) had been passed down from her grandmother. With this woman, I embarked upon a spiritual training in the European shamanic tradition and was initiated on this path in 1987. The word *shaman* comes from the language of the Tungus tribe in Siberia. It has since been used by anthropologists and scholars to describe practitioners from diverse cultures worldwide who act as intermediaries between the physical and spiritual worlds by communing with Spirit for healing, guidance, and the benefit of their communities. In shamanic cultures it is accepted that plants have a spiritual nature, just like humans, animals, rocks, clouds, and all living things do. Therefore, this training encouraged my spiritual view of plants and helped me to integrate a shamanic approach with modern-day herbal medicine. Since that time I have practiced as a clinical herbalist, a healer, and a ceremonialist, blending my shamanic background with contemporary herbal medicine and flower essence therapy.

I was very inspired by the pioneering work with nature spirits at Findhorn in Scotland and Perelandra in the United States. In 1992 on a visit to Findhorn, I attended a lecture on flower essences by an Irishman who at the time was working in the Findhorn gardens. This led me to visit Ireland the following year, intending to do a flower essence course with

---

*In Europe the terms *hedgewitch* and *Wise Woman* refer to a local wise person who uses his or her knowledge of herbalism and natural magic to help the community. Some see this as similar to the Ovates (healers, seers, and diviners) who represent a stream of Druidry (along with Bards and Druids) that seemed to mostly disappear by around the sixth century. It is reasonable to suggest that, rather than abandoning their healing skills with the advent of Christianity, the Celtic Druid Ovates instead went underground and through the word-of-mouth tradition later became the hedgewitches. Philip Carr-Gomm (Chief of the Order of Bards Ovates and Druids in the UK) discusses this point in his book *DruidCraft: The Magic of Wicca and Druidry* (see the bibliography).

this man. The trip changed my life. Despite having Irish ancestors, I had never been to Ireland before and had never considered moving here. Yet as I flew into Dublin and saw the land beneath the plane, I experienced a profound response in my body and knew that this land was my home. I realized I was being called to live and work in Ireland. I traveled to Donegal asking Spirit for guidance, and it became crystal clear that Ireland was where my family and I needed to live. On one occasion that weekend, I sat with my hands on a huge boulder in a forest, asking to be shown a sign of confirmation. To my amazement this enormous boulder began to vibrate visibly, with such force that it reminded me of a spin drier, and I thought it might take off.

By the time I returned to my family in England, I knew without doubt that we had to move to Ireland. This was a total surprise for my husband Steve and sons, then ages five and three. Several weeks later our entire family traveled to Ireland to see how it felt. Thankfully Steve was in full agreement about moving here. That week we planned to tour the country, asking to be guided to where we were meant to be. A man in Kerry told us about a house that had belonged to Biddy Early (a well-known nineteenth-century herbalist in County Clare) that was up for sale and how the owners wanted to sell it to another herbalist. Surely this was a sign we should follow. On arriving in Feakle we knew this area was calling us. Biddy Early had led us to Feakle, and while we did not end up buying her house, she showed us where to look. It took another eighteen months for us to sell our house in England and for me to wind down my herbal practice. Finally we set off through the snow in the early spring of 1995, the four of us and our belongings in an old rickety jeep, heading for County Clare. Spirit was sending us on an adventure!

We came to Ireland with the intention of working with Nature to co-create a place of beauty, a sanctuary where the plant world would be honored and where people could come for healing, to learn about plants, and to experience the spirit of the plants and the Spirit that resides within all beings. We hoped that in this sanctuary people would feel the sense of connectedness that exists between all forms of life—mineral, plant, animal, and human, believing as we did that if we truly recognize Spirit within all beings, we are much more likely to care for the planet and all Her beings.

Initially we rented a mobile home, and later a house in the village, while we searched for our new home. I set up my herbal practice and was delighted to immerse myself in the innate spirituality and connection to the land that I experience in the people here. I love the land of Ireland, and from my first visit I was struck by how accessible the nature spirits are. For someone working with plant spirits it can be paradise! Our quest was to find a place that could be our home, healing center, garden, and plant sanctuary. After more than two years of searching, and some bitter disappointments, I began to wonder if perhaps Spirit's plan for us was to not have our own place. I knew this area was where we had to live and work but maybe we weren't meant to buy a house or land. Finally I did a ceremony on the dark moon to let go of expectation, while surrendering to Spirit and committing to doing whatever was required to adhere to Spirit's plan. A few days later our neighbor told us about Derrynagittah. When we visited here we knew straight away that this was to be our home. Spirit powerfully reinforced the message as I was thrown to the ground by the shock from an electric fence, feeling as if I had been struck with a huge piece of wood. Lying stunned on the ground, I realized the land was telling me to wake up and take notice, showing me that this was where we should be and that we needed to *act*. It was a definite wake-up call. The sale went through in a matter of days.

Derrynagittah is the name of this townland (a small division of land particular to Ireland) and in Gaelic means "the oak wood of the left-handed people." We are blessed to live on twenty-nine acres of magical land in the Grainey Valley in east Clare. Here we have restored the old farmhouse as our home, and built a clinic for my herbal practice and medicine making. We have two outdoor temples where I conduct group and personal ceremonies: a medicine-wheel herb garden and a stone-walled plant labyrinth. We have also built a ten-sided sound temple that provides an indoor group ceremonial space, dedicated to plants and sound healing as well as other appropriate ceremonies. It is within these sacred temples that our plant initiations take place.

In 1998 I met Arwyn DreamWalker from Arizona, a medicine woman of Native American and Irish descent, and a master teacher, healer, dreamer, and seer. She is a lineage carrier for the Dineh people (Navaho) and teaches the Beauty Way tradition and other teachings passed to her by Navaho Grandfather Tom Wilson. Walking a path of beauty involves living in harmony with Nature and honoring all life as sacred. The Beauty Way can be viewed as a path of heart, of knowing who you are and following your heart with integrity among your people, family, and community. DreamWalker's work holds at its heart a deep devotion to the sacred and she has profoundly influenced my life with her compassion and impeccable teachings. In 2010 I completed a ten-year apprenticeship with this remarkable teacher. Working with DreamWalker has helped me to recognize and honor the sacred in all of life, and to know and walk my soul's dream. Part of my sacred offering includes opening doorways for others, so they can know their own sacred relationship with plants.

The labyrinth is another major focus of our work at Derrynagittah. In 2000, after reading about labyrinths in *Network* magazine, I received strong guidance to build a stone-walled plant labyrinth (see color plate 1). At that time I knew very little about labyrinths and the idea of taking on yet another building project with our already stretched resources seemed rather ridiculous. Yet the urging from Spirit was strong and could not be ignored. The building of the labyrinth was a slow process that challenged us in ways we could never have imagined. It seemed a miracle when it was finally completed in 2003.

A labyrinth is a powerful and ancient archetypal symbol. Labyrinths carry the energy of the Divine Feminine. They represent wholeness, balancing male and female, yin and yang, and are considered symbols of the Goddess and of fertility. The labyrinth at Derrynagittah is a classic seven-ring labyrinth, which is an ancient design. The rings correspond to the first seven energy centers (light wheels or chakras) in the body and are planted with appropriate herbs and flowers for each light wheel. The center of the labyrinth corresponds to the higher light wheels and is a place of transformation. Walking the labyrinth can be seen as a pilgrimage to the center of oneself. The labyrinth here is dedicated to Shekinah as the embodiment of the Divine Feminine.* The labyrinth is a gateway that links with the earth energy grid or song lines of the Earth and connects us to the stars and planets. As well as offering transformation for ourselves and our communities, a labyrinth can be walked and worked with to bring benefit to Grandmother Earth.

At the time of building the labyrinth I had no clear idea of how it was to be used. However, soon after its completion Spirit told me that it now needed a group of people to work with. So at the Autumn Equinox of 2003 I held a group ceremony for the Fire Festival and invited an assorted collection of people to join me for a so-called labyrinth study group.† They had no idea what they were coming to. Most of these people had not met each other before and some I hardly knew myself. However, this group continued to meet at every Fire Festival and quickly blossomed into a thriving community that participated in a range of activities, including our early plant diets.

The idea of dieting native plants had been with me for many years and once I was in Ireland I had a strong sense that the native plants were calling out to be dieted in a ceremonial way. One of the difficulties in tracing our own traditional European plant diets has been the loss of our oral tradition, a particular result of witch burnings in which so many shamans were wiped out or went underground. I knew I was waiting for further instructions.

Without a living teacher or guide, and only sketchy information about European plant diets, I was forced back on my own experience and the guidance from my helpers in Spirit. I did my best to listen to the plants to know what was being called for. With visiting shamans I took part in plant diets with nonnative plants and these plants urged me to go deeper, to reconnect with an old way of working, and to bring it forward into the present day—to *wake up and remember*. With this in mind, in 2008 I decided to visit Peru to work with a shaman in the

---

*The goddess Shekinah represents the Divine Feminine. She is the manifestation of the Wisdom Goddess of the Kabbalah, the Old Testament, and Merkavah mysticism.

†Holding ceremony at the Fire Festivals is a way of honoring the Earth and aligning with the cycles of Nature.

Amazon, dieting with the native plants of South America. Thus, I went to Peru with the intention of remembering the ancient European ways of plant dieting so that I could offer this to the people on behalf of the plants of Ireland.

My trip to Peru marked a major turning point and taught me many things. Upon returning home to Ireland, I was ready to start dieting the medicinal plants growing around me. I intended to begin by experimenting on myself, however I had not anticipated the enthusiasm of the labyrinth study group. Once they heard what I was intending to do, they unanimously volunteered to take part. Thus it was that in 2008 I began holding plant diet ceremonies for the group at Derrynagittah.

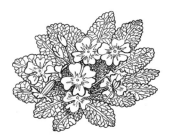

*Primrose*

Primrose was the first plant we dieted. This choice of plant arose primarily from our work with the labyrinth. During our ongoing dreamings with the labyrinth, members of the group had been receiving information that the flowers are keys that open gateways in the labyrinth and the labyrinth, in turn, is a key that opens gateways to consciousness. It was following a night of such images in 2005 that during an herbal consultation, a patient, who was also a traditional storyteller, told me the story of the Key Flower, which portrays a beautiful flower as a magical key that unlocks the door to wondrous treasures. As the tale unfolded, I realized that the story contained important information for our ongoing work with the labyrinth and with the plants. The resonance between the message of this story and our own experiences was very strong. This is the story as it was told (this version is thought to have originated in Scotland), with thanks to Ruth Marshall.

### The Story of the Key Flower

*Long ago atop a green hill in Wales, a shepherd watched his flock grazing. In the grass at his feet he noticed the most beautiful flower he had ever seen, which he picked and put in his buttonhole, enjoying its sweet scent. That afternoon he led the sheep up the hill. There on the hillside he came upon a stone door that he had never seen before. He wondered if somehow he'd gotten lost, but no, looking around he saw this was indeed the old familiar valley where the sheep had always grazed.*

*The shepherd tried opening the stone door but it wouldn't budge. Then he noticed it had a little keyhole. Looking down at his buttonhole, he saw that the shape of the flower's petals were remarkably akin to that of the keyhole. Chancing that the flower might fit, he tried it in the hole. To his surprise it fit perfectly and when he turned the flower, the stone door opened.*

*You might expect it to be dark and chilly inside that hill but it wasn't. From the center of the hill there shone a Light that glistened like sunrise on a lake. The shepherd stepped inside and walked toward it, where he found all manner of treasures: mounds of shimmering gold and shining silver, heaps of bright emeralds, rubies, sapphires, and pearls. The poor astonished shepherd could barely catch his breath for such riches were beyond imagining. He thought of his loved ones waiting back at the cottage and began stuffing his pockets to the brim, taking off his socks and using them as pouches and using his wool cap as a sack.*

*Hurriedly he set out for home. The weight of the riches was great upon him but his gait was light, nonetheless, for he imagined the joy on his loved ones' faces when he shared with them the dazzling gems.*

*The farther he got from the hill, the lighter the load seemed to grow and soon he could no longer feel the weight of it, so he stopped to check his pockets and pouches. To his great dismay, they were not filled with jewels nor riches, but with leaves, crumbly dry leaves, the likes of which he would rake up and toss on the compost heap. The shepherd turned his pockets inside out, and the bits of dry leaves blew away on the wind. He trudged home puzzling over the day, trying to make sense of what had happened.*

*When the shepherd got home, he wanted to tell the story of the Key*

*Flower, the stone door, and the riches inside the hill, but when he tried*
*to speak of it his throat grew dry and his thoughts scattered. He knew*
*whatever he said would sound foolish, so he kept quiet.*

*In the days and weeks to come he often searched for the stone door*
*but he never found it. He scanned the grassy hills for another Key Flower,*
*though none was ever to be found.*

*It wasn't until much later, sitting at the fireside one night, that he*
*decided to tell his tale. In his mind's eye he saw it all with great clarity as if*
*it had been yesterday. The thoughts formed freely in his mind and flowed*
*from his lips like a river. Afterward his loved ones remarked what a fine*
*story it was, and that he was a good teller of tales. He told them it was all*
*true, every last detail, and they scoffed, "What a rascal you are."*

*As the years passed by, the memory of that afternoon stayed bright*
*within him. Even as a very old man, thinking about it brought a smile to*
*his lips.*

This story reinforces the message of flowers being keys to expanded awareness. By appreciating the beauty of the flower, the shepherd is taken through a gateway and shown incredible riches. However, on finding what appears to be the treasure, he forgets about the flower and gives more value to the gold and jewels before him. We are urged to recognize what is truly valuable in life. It is only by valuing Nature that we can receive Her abundant gifts.

With further research, I discovered that one of the traditional European names for Primrose is Key Flower.* In Germany the popular name is *Schusselblume* (Key Flower) and in Dutch it is *Sleutelbloem* (Key Flower). It is also commonly known as Heaven's Key (*Himmelschussel* in German), St. Peter's Key, St. Peter's Wort (in England), and Herbe de Saint Pierre (in France). Similar Key Flower stories exist in many different cultures and traditions. In the traditional stories of Germany, Primrose is often seen as a gift from the gods that points the way to hidden treasure. Finding Primrose is considered auspicious, especially if it is discovered still flowering

---

*Key Flower is often used interchangeably for both Primrose and Cowslip.

on Christmas Day or Shrove Tuesday. Having found this flower, a female deity often thought to be Freya, Norse Goddess of Love and Beauty, is said to appear to the finder with a key hidden in her crown. The key points to, and unlocks, the door where the treasure is hidden.

Primrose legends of other countries such as England and Switzerland tell of how a young shepherd finds a golden yellow flower that leads to a hidden doorway in a rock, in which there is hidden treasure. On finding the treasure, however, the boy leaves the flower on the floor within the rock, and as he leaves he pays no heed to a voice calling out to him, "Do not forget the best thing!" Consequently he is no longer able to get to the treasure.

## THE PRIMROSES OF ISLAY

Another development in my relationship with Primrose came in June 2007. I received a call from an old friend from England, Eleanor, whom I hadn't spoken to in years. Eleanor revealed that she was now living in Scotland and wanted to talk to me about labyrinths. She told me she had bought one thousand acres of forest on the Isle of Islay in Scotland, where she and her family were planning to set up a bed and breakfast. She had also been asked by Spirit to build a labyrinth on her land, which was why she was contacting me, looking for advice. Eleanor is a medium and has received Spirit messages all her life, so she is well used to acting on Spirit's guidance. We spoke a little about labyrinths and later on that day she called me back, saying she had just gone for a walk on her land and Spirit had given her precise instructions for a ceremony she needed to do at 7:00 p.m. on the following day. This was a big surprise to her because, while she has years of experience as a medium, it is not her usual practice to do ceremonies or anything shamanic.

Eleanor was told "to go out to the highest mountain on her land, from which it is possible to see the land of Ireland, and to place a rowan stake in the ground." She was instructed to "call on the Celtic Druids to release the energy, to bless the stake, and to open the portals." She was asked to call on the "four Nordic horsemen from North, South, East, and West to take the Celtic Druidic forces of healing and Light into the North, South, East, and

West." They were to "ride with them across the sea to Ireland, bring them to Clare to reclaim all that was, to open up and erase the barriers of ancient and modern." Eleanor was told to inform me of this so that I could do all that was necessary to prepare for the arrival of these energies. She was told that the energies needed to be received in the labyrinth and then sent out around the Earth. While we were speaking on the telephone, all I was seeing were images of Primroses, so I asked Eleanor if the Primrose held any significance for her. She told me that there were Primroses flowering everywhere on her land. I asked her to send me some Primroses from her land so that I could plant them in the labyrinth or wherever they called to go. In fact they were planted in various places—some in the third ring of the labyrinth (relating to the third chakra or third light wheel, which is yellow in color), some at other places on our land, and some at other sacred sites in Ireland.

With regard to the Nordic horsemen, I wasn't entirely sure who they were but my guidance was encouraging me to welcome them, so we gathered in the center of the labyrinth at 7:00 p.m. to receive and anchor these ancient Druidic energies. I called also for the blessings of Primrose and I have no doubt that Primrose played, and continues to play, her own role in helping the flow of Earth's energies. The Nordic horsemen carried on with their journey to the four directions, spreading the energies and helping to forge and deepen the ongoing connection between our labyrinth and the labyrinth Eleanor has now built on Islay. Only later did I realize the horsemen's connection to a different labyrinth in Sweden that I have worked with regularly since 2004. Over time, this work has opened my awareness to the powerful energy channel that pours through Ireland from the Nordic countries.

## LOUGH GUR

One of the sacred sites where we planted the Islay Primroses was at Lough Gur in County Limerick. This is an ancient site with a beautiful lake, stone circles, and a variety of standing stones. There was a clear message that the energies received in Clare needed to be anchored at Lough Gur, and from there they would spread over to continental Europe.

It is said that Lough Gur was formed by the goddess Áine who appears there in different forms as mermaid, young woman, and hag. As mermaid, she rises from her traditional home beneath the sacred waters of the lake. As maiden, she empowers the human custodians of the land. As hag, she defends her realm. Áine's son, Gearóid Iarla, is said to ride across the surface of the Lough Gur every seven years on a milk-white horse with silver shoes. According to legend he is destined to do this until the silver shoes are worn away, at which time he will ride forth and gain freedom for all of Ireland. The freedom that is promised here is the freedom of Spirit, the dawn of a new consciousness. Another legend holds that once every seven years the enchanted lake dries up and the sacred tree at the bottom of the lake can be seen covered with a green cloth. An old woman (Áine as hag) keeps watch from beneath the cloth. She is knitting, recreating the fabric of life, stitch by stitch, with intentionality and purpose.

This image of Áine knitting the fabric of life is consistent with an image we can relate to in our present time. The following is a message received via Tom Kenyon* from the Hathors in 2009, reminding us how we can choose to create an entirely new reality:

The fabric of your old realities is being unwound at the same time that new realities are being woven. This is, indeed, an odd state. And what we wish to convey most clearly is that you have the innate power and ability to weave new realities for yourself, new freedoms of mind and spirit, regardless of what is happening around you.

Given what we have perceived as Primrose's power to open higher states of consciousness, it is entirely fitting to have planted Primroses at Lough Gur, where Áine knits and waits for the time when the silver horse shoes will be worn away and the milk white horse bearing her son will ride forth to awaken freedom within the heart of Ireland. When we went to

---

*Tom Kenyon is a sound healer and teacher who channels messages from the Hathors. This message is extracted from *The Holon of Ascension*, January 28, 2009. See www .tomkenyon.com. At the time of receiving this material, the labyrinth group had been on another recent pilgrimage to Lough Gur and the imagery in the message was particularly resonant with our experiences of Áine.

Lough Gur in October 2007 to plant the Islay Primroses, there was a green moss covering the land, which recalled for us the fabric of Áine's endeavor. As we planted Primroses, dragonflies came and circled around us, speaking to us of transformation* and reminding us of the presence of faeries.

In October 2007, while I was on an inner journey to meet the goddess Éiru, the goddess informed me that Primroses could help to clear her song lines. Éiru (a triple goddess with her sisters Banbha and Fódla) is often considered the personification of Ireland, and she is seen as the Goddess of Sovereignty. She said we should plant more at other sacred sites and that they act like acupuncture needles for the land and Her energies.

You can understand why, in 2008, Primrose was my first chosen plant to diet. When I came to prepare for the Primrose diet, the first book I looked in, the herbal of English herbalist John Gerard (1545–1611), gave me the following piece of information:

> A practitioner of London who was famous for curing the phrensie, after he had performed his cure by the due observation of physic, accustomed every yeare in the moneth of May to dyet his Patients after this manner: Take the leaves and flowers of Primrose, boile them a little in fountaine water, and in some rose and Betony waters, adding thereto sugar, pepper, salt, and butter, which being strained he gave them to drinke thereof, first and last.[†]

This means they took Primrose to drink morning and night. What a wonderful affirmation of our work!

---

*Dragonflies are associated with transformation because they start their life in the water and end it as creatures of land and sky. In Ireland, faeries are said to disguise themselves as dragonflies and their true identity can be revealed by rubbing one's eyelids with a Primrose.

[†]John Gerard, *Generall Historie of Plants* (London: Islip, Norton & Whitakers, 1636), 179.

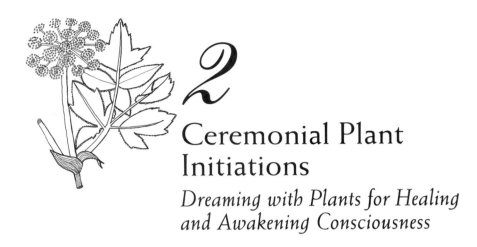

# 2

# Ceremonial Plant Initiations

*Dreaming with Plants for Healing and Awakening Consciousness*

> *Great Spirit, may I always remember*
> *That everything in life is Sacred.*
> *May I live my life*
> *As a walking prayer.*

Ceremonial plant dieting is an ancient method of honoring and connecting with a plant. The ceremonial process opens gateways to spiritual realms and facilitates powerful development at physical, emotional, mental, and spiritual levels. As mentioned in the introduction, this type of plant dieting involves the sacred and conscious ingestion of a plant for healing and transformation. A relationship is formed whereby the plant acts as one who initiates the human into the next level of awakening. In this book we will explore various methods of creating and deepening that relationship. Here, we experience plants as conscious beings who have much to teach us. We receive many gifts from the plants and we acknowledge that our relationships are reciprocal; we must, therefore, also give back.

As we shift into a new era, we humans are being offered many new gateways to higher consciousness. Plant dieting is one such opening. It easily gives us access to higher dimensions and creative worlds within us, and it can retune our brains to receive new frequencies. In addition, a plant diet helps us to develop a close relationship with a plant and indeed this can change our relationship with the entire plant world.

Being initiated by a plant offers the possibility of merging with its consciousness. Thus, we can experience the connectedness of all life and thereby access Oneness through the plant world. The physical ingestion of the plant helps to ground and integrate new levels of consciousness into the physical body. It helps the body to adjust to a higher vibration and can radically change our cellular structure. By ingesting a plant, the body charges itself like a battery from the energies of that plant. Ultimately, the plant may become part of our cells, filling us with energy and with the potential to offer healing for others.

A plant diet can support, strengthen, and heal us on all levels of our being. By doing this, these diets facilitate deep and lasting transformation. If we are willing, we can not only receive a whole new blueprint but also change our physical structure and anchor the new patterns firmly in our cellular makeup. A plant diet can help us to wake up and remember who we are, connecting us with the plants, the Earth, and the entire Universe. Essentially, this kind of plant diet offers an initiation, facilitating the flowering of human potential and inviting us to truly live as sacred humans. Initiation involves a personal test—in order to grow and move forward we are challenged to face our deepest fears and to accept the challenges life brings. Ceremony is central to this process, reinforcing the sacredness of the plant world and reminding us of how we can be in service to life.

## NONPSYCHOACTIVE PLANT DIETS

In modern Western culture, plant diets are often associated with plants known as Teacher Plants, Master Plants, or Plants of Vision. These are generally psychoactive plants like Ayahausca,* Datura, Sacred Mushrooms, Peyote, and many other plants and fungi that offer visionary experiences and are described as opening gateways to higher consciousness. *Psychoactive, psycho-pharmaceutical,* and *psychotropic* are terms used to describe a chemical substance that crosses the blood-brain barrier and acts primarily upon the central nervous system, affecting brain function and resulting in changes in perception, mood, consciousness, behavior, and cognition.

The experiences described in this book are of plant diets taken with nonpsychoactive plants. These include plants such as Primrose, Dandelion, Elder, and Dog Rose, all common medicinal plants growing in our hedgerows and not typically well known for their consciousness-raising effects (see color plate 2). Our experience has shown us that these nonpsychoactive native plants have their own potential to open gateways to higher consciousness, and to invoke the mystical. I would contest that these plants, therefore, deserve to be classed as *entheogenic* in that they "generate the Divine within." This term is usually reserved to refer to psychoactive substances only.

In my experience, while not chemically psychoactive, the plants we are dieting expand awareness and facilitate direct communion with Spirit. They can induce visions and enable us to explore other dimensions. Perhaps, when approached with honor and reverence, all plants can behave in this way. Certainly they differ from Master Plants in terms of character and behavior. Along with their strong personalities, I have found that certain Master Plants act as designers and choreographers, sometimes setting a template for other plants to follow. The nonpsychoactive plants tend to be gentler and less forceful, but they are coming forward at this time with outstanding gifts to offer the world. In this book I aim to demonstrate the healing and consciousness-raising potential of these plants by presenting a qualitative analysis of our personal experiences during the plant-diet ceremonies in

---

*The brew commonly known as Ayahuasca is made up of more than one plant. To become a visionary medicine for humans, the Ayahuasca vine (*Banisteriopsis caapi*) is boiled in water with at least one other ingredient. One widely used plant for this purpose is Chacruna (*Psychotria viridis*). Other ingredients may be added, such as Tobacco or Datura, depending on who is making the medicine and for what purpose it will be used.

Derrynagittah (and, in one instance, Vermont). I am sharing my methods in the hope that you may be inspired to do your own dieting with some of these plants or with other common plants or trees native to your home. This is an area that calls for further study and I look forward to hearing the results of others' research. These plants are already on our doorsteps, sustainable and accessible. They need no air miles to travel here and I believe they are actively encouraging us to connect to their realm in a sacred manner.

## CEREMONIAL PLANT DIETS IN HOLISTIC HERBAL TREATMENT

As an herbalist in a plant-based healing practice, I work with herbs and flower essences and I call on the spirits of the plants to help my patients. I aim to treat body, emotions, mind, and spirit in a balanced way. To do this I need to draw on the most appropriate tools and methods to address the individual needs of a client. This requires working with the whole plant for the whole person. In this context, I love the holistic nature of the plant diets. In these ceremonial diets the whole plant is called upon to make an elixir that is our sacrament. Working with these elixirs brings together all the healing aspects of the plant and represents a truly holistic approach. During a plant diet, sacred ceremony is central to the initiation experience.

What do I mean by ceremony? A sacred ceremony connects the physical and spiritual realms. It is a way to acknowledge and deepen our spirituality, our connections to ourselves and to all of life. The physical form and structure of a ceremony allow us to access other dimensions through our intention (more on intention in chapter 3). A ceremony is strong and authentic when it focuses our energies, connects us with our higher self, and lifts us into states of expanded consciousness.

By working with plants in ceremony, we can experience life in ways that are not normally accessible in everyday consciousness. Working in this way brings an influx of beneficial energy and helps give clarity and form to our intentions. It gives us a sacred space where mystery can manifest. Ceremony does not have to be complicated. It does not have to come from any particular tradition or religion. The ceremonies I conduct are spiritual rather than religious. They are intended to be inclusive of all. Ceremony may be carried out alone or with a group of people. We are free to create whatever kind of ceremony we need that expresses our heartfelt desire.

Working with plants in ceremony is a way of honoring both the plants and the Spirit in all beings. It is a way of being in service to the plant world. This last statement may seem strange when the plants give us so much during a plant diet. Yet in my experience the plants love to give, and therefore we serve them by treating them with gratitude and respect and by facilitating their giving. Respect is crucial and this includes recognizing that we are neither separate from, nor superior to, plants. Our lives are no more or less important than theirs. This is a two-way exchange of energy. We receive the gifts of the plants and we also need to give back to them. How can we give back? One way to be of service is to make good use of the gifts we are given. This may include passing these gifts on to others, whether through healing, teaching, or other forms of expression. We can also take the time to ask the plants what they would like, and be sure to follow up on this information. Actions we take for the plant world can be diverse, ranging from activities such as making changes in our lives, growing a certain plant, or creating a piece of artwork to engaging in community activism, such as protecting a forest or campaigning for the environment. Ultimately, these ceremonies need to serve the wider community and our intention must always be to bring blessings to others.

## A TURNING POINT FOR THE PLANET

We stand now at an important turning point in the history of our planet. Ancient prophecies from the Mayans, various Native American tribes, and many others describe planet Earth as entering a new phase. This is the dawning of a new world (or the world of the fifth sun as the Hopis have called it). The planet is evolving and all of life on Earth has an opportunity to evolve along with Her. In each one of us humans, this is an opportunity to make a paradigm shift and evolve in consciousness— to live in our hearts, to awaken spiritually, and to accept the reality of higher dimensions. Currently on our planet much is being cleansed and released as Earth goes through Her own evolutionary process. Human actions continue to damage the planet and the effects can be very painful. It is easy to succumb to fear in these challenging times. And yet, unity consciousness—the awareness of our interconnectedness—is flooding the planet, together with an abundance of help, both spiritual and physical.

Plants are among those beings offering key assistance, and this is an area where plant initiations are particularly valuable, since they make this assistance accessible. Plants seem to be evolving ahead of most humans and can lead the way for us. They can help us with the rapid expansion of human consciousness that is possible at this time. Plants are our very ancient relatives. The first plants emerged on our planet at some time between 2,100 and 1,200 million years ago. These ancient plants started as algae living in water and began to move onto dry land around 470 million years ago. Plants have continued to evolve, moving from mosses to ferns and eventually to seed plants (heterospories) and flowering plants (angiosperms). Flowering plants rapidly overtook our planet, and Darwin described their origin as an "abominable mystery," since the speed of their arrival did not fit with his idea that the emergence of new species could only take place very gradually. Current scientific research still considers the emergence of seed plants to be somewhat of a mystery. It has been postulated that flowering plants were able to change the world to suit their own needs, and the study of epigenetics may give further clues.*

Whatever the answer, evolution continues and we humans need to sign up fast. Viewed from a perspective of wholeness, our lack of human awareness can be seen to inhibit the overall evolutionary process. Plants offer to initiate us into more connected levels of being, while acting as a stabilizing force that helps us to hold and integrate new frequencies. This can have a knock-on effect. The more we raise our human consciousness and restore the relationship between humans and plants, the easier it is for

---

*Frank Berendse and Marten Scheffer, "The Angiosperm Radiation Revisited, an Ecological Explanation for Darwin's 'Abominable Mystery,'" *Ecology Letters* 26 (9) (2009): 865–72.

the plant world and the nature spirits to flourish in their full beauty and fulfill their potential.

## The Age of Flowers and the Evolution of Plants

From the teachings of Arwyn DreamWalker, I have learned that according to the Maya we are moving through what is called the Age of Flowers, described as a time when the flower devas* would bring special gifts to help the world with purification and transformation. It is said the plants will bring powerful messages of deep healing, bringing us hope and the ability to awaken to all that we are. Others have been reporting new plants appearing on the planet and previously extinct plants are said to be returning. For example, in 2012 a team of scientists in Russia successfully regenerated seeds of *Silene stenophylla* from fruit that had been frozen for 30,000 years, according to radiocarbon dating. The fruits and seeds had been recovered from an ancient rodent burrow in the Siberian permafrost.[†]

In Ireland, I find more and more plants are emerging that have transformed and are carrying new qualities. My experience is that these transformed plants are behaving as pioneers and leading the way not only for other plants but for all of life, including the human species. For instance, St. John's Wort is carrying what I perceive as a new form of Light that can help us make the transition to living in the heart (see chapter 11 for more details on this Light). I also find that plants and crystals are combining more and more often to work together for the purpose of spiritual evolution. What I experience in Ireland may be the same process that has been reported by holistic health practitioner Merri Walters at the Great Lakes in Canada, where she describes encountering plants that have "already gone through the transition."[‡] I imagine this is happening worldwide.

---

*Deva* is a Sanskrit word meaning "shining one." The devas hold the archetypal pattern and plan for all forms around us. The devic kingdom represents the overlighting intelligence or the "architects" for the physical bodies of life forms (animal, vegetable, mineral, and human). They direct the energy needed to materialize form.

[†]S. Yashina, S. Gubin, and S. Maksimovich, et al., "Regeneration of Whole Fertile Plants From 30,000-year-old Fruit Tissue Buried in Siberian Permafrost," *Proceedings of the National Academy of Sciences USA* 10 (1073) (2012): pnas. 11183861.

[‡]See www.sacredessences.com for the work of Merri Walters.

We are fortunate to be living in these exciting times and I am constantly filled with gratitude when I see the generosity of the plants. At this time of Earth's evolution, it is essential for us to align our intent with the direction and purpose of Spirit. The Earth knows what is needed far better than most humans do. She is in the process of birthing a new way and a rapid quickening is taking place. We have to wake up and listen, let go of our ego control, allow ourselves to be guided, and act accordingly. It is time to remember who we really are and why we are here. The plant diets put us in touch with Grandmother Earth and can help us to hear Her and our true selves. They can give us a direct experience of other realms and dimensions.

To many of us, these times can seem overwhelming. We worry that anything we try to do will be too little, too late and that as a race, humans are incapable of so much transformation. I know these feelings but I also know that we have chosen to be here on Earth at this time. I choose to believe that anything is possible and that it is up to each of us to co-create a new dream of beauty. The plant world comes with a generous heart, offering to dream with us and to help us find a new way forward.

In the next two chapters, I describe my own methods of developing and carrying out ceremonial plant initiations and give guidelines for you to design your own. My methods have arisen from my own background and life experience and by being in co-creation with the spirit world. The exact form of each ceremony varies depending on the plant being dieted, the people present, the timing, and many other factors. Appendix 2 on pages 279–80 gives a simplified format to further assist you in carrying out your own plant initiations. Appendix 4 on pages 286–87 describes specially recorded music and meditations that can be freely downloaded and incorporated into your ceremonial plant diets at audio.innertraditions .com/saplin.

The suggestions in this book are for guidance and inspiration. They are not intended as rigid instructions. Developing a ceremonial plant diet simply requires that you recognize the sacredness of plants and honor the Spirit that exists in all beings. The ceremony can take whatever form you choose, but it must have meaning for you personally. Successive chapters take you on a journey through the Wheel of the Year, describing plants that we have dieted at Derrynagittah, methods of preparation, and our experiences at these ceremonies.

The gifts of a plant diet are accessible to anyone who approaches the work with an open heart and an attitude of gratitude and respect for the plant world. The plants offer us a deep, nourishing connection with all of life. They offer to help us remember who we are so that we can fulfill our destinies. These gifts are available to every one of us, and the process may be much easier than you think.

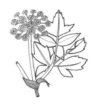

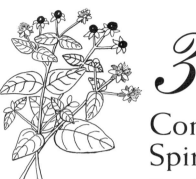

# 3

# Connecting with the Spirit of Plants

*Step-by-Step Instructions for Connecting with Plant Consciousness*

*Hey! Magnificent Green Beings,*
*You who spread your mantle of Beauty*
*Over the surface of the Grandmother!*
*Beloved Ones I long to be with you,*
*To feel your presence, within and without,*
*To lose myself in your Greenness.*
*Let me travel in your cells as you travel in mine,*
*Welcoming you in as I give of myself,*
*Experiencing our Oneness.*

*I*n order to carry out your own plant initiation ceremonies you will want to have an authentic way to connect with the consciousness of plants. If this is new for you, this chapter presents simple methods to help you connect with the spirit of plants. If you are already experienced with plant communication, you can either skip this chapter or perhaps you may discover some additional ways to help deepen your plant relationships.

I feel at home in the plant world and many plants are close friends. Some of them are more acquaintances and some take longer to get to know than others. This is normal. Basically I relate to plants in the same kind of way that I relate to humans. Always remember that plants have consciousness. Treat them with respect. Talk to them. This does not have to be out loud, although they do respond to our voices. They are also much cleverer at telepathy than most humans! You may find it similar to the way you communicate with a beloved cat or dog or other animal.

Plants easily connect through feelings. Whatever you are feeling has an impact on the plants around you. If you approach them feeling love and gratitude, awe and wonder, they will certainly respond. These feelings cause your heart to open, and having an open heart is the easiest way I know to connect with plants. Simply relax and enjoy the beauty of the plants around you. If necessary in the beginning stages of your time with plants, tell yourself you are playing a game and pretend that you are communicating with the plants. Trick your mind and allow your imagination to lead you.

## ✿ EXERCISE TO CONNECT WITH THE SPIRIT OF A LIVING PLANT

1. Relax and trust that you can indeed make a connection with a plant spirit. It is only the civilized human mind that tends to make things complicated. Not only is this easy, it's fun!
2. Set a clear intention to connect with the spirit of a plant.
3. Go to where the plants are. Typically this will be outside, but you could also meet a plant indoors. It is often helpful to bring a notebook and pencil or crayons so you can record your findings and do some drawing. Repeat steps 1 and 2. Become aware of the beauty around you. Engender feelings of wonder and gratitude. Open your heart and become childlike. When your heart is open, the plants can easily attune to you. You will very likely feel a kind of magnetic pull to a certain plant or group of plants. They love it when we genuinely reach out to them, and they will usually beckon you. Let yourself be guided to whoever is calling. Sometimes there will be many plants calling at once and you have to make a decision who to go to!

4. Approach the plant, expressing your genuine appreciation. Plants respond to your thoughts and feelings, and they also respond to the sound of your voice if you speak out loud. Be aware that you are entering the energy field of this being. Plants, like humans, are surrounded by a biomagnetic energy field known as the aura. You may find that you can see, sense, or feel the plant's auric field. Are you aware of the colors of its aura? Can you sense the energy around the plant? What is the flow of this energy? Don't worry if you can't sense anything initially. Simply know that this energy field exists. Become aware of sound and the general atmosphere around the plant. Are there bees humming or birds singing? Perhaps you can hear traffic noise or human voices. You are entering into the dreamtime of the plant, and whatever you perceive is part of that dream.

5. Introduce yourself to the plant, explain your intention, and ask permission to come closer and spend time with it, just as you would if meeting a human. Listen to how your heart feels to know if you have permission. This inner knowing is often more obvious than you may think. If you suddenly feel very cold, unwell, unhappy, or experience any sense that says "no" for you, then now is probably not the time to proceed with this plant. This could be for a variety of reasons. Perhaps you are approaching with the wrong attitude. Alternatively, it may simply not be the right timing due to any number of other factors. In most cases this is unlikely to occur, and you can proceed to enter into the field of consciousness of the plant.

6. Examine the plant with your outer senses, spending time experiencing each physical sense:

   ᕁ First, look at the appearance of the plant. Study the shapes, colors, number of petals, and formation of the leaves. How does it grow? Is it spreading or compact? Is it reaching out to the sun or resting in the shade? Does it have its feet in water or is it in a dry area? Is it a lone plant growing on its own or is it in a large group? Is it growing with plants of other species? What is its community? You may want to draw the plant at this stage. Making a detailed drawing requires that you really *see* the plant and pay attention to small details. All of this gives you information about the plant and helps you to connect with it and know it better.

- Now connect with the plant through touch. Feel the texture. Does it remind you of anything? Touch the plant like a lover. Feel it through your fingertips, stroking and caressing it, patting it, or running your hand along the leaves or stem.

- Smell the plant. What is its aroma and what does this invoke?

- It may be appropriate (please be sure it's not poisonous!) to taste a little of the plant. You can touch it with your tongue or lick the plant. You may even be invited to ingest some of the plant. How does it taste? What does the taste invoke? Is there a difference of taste in different parts of your mouth? How do you feel after swallowing?

- Now listen to the plant. What can you hear? Are its leaves rustling in the breeze or do its seedpods rattle? What do the sounds remind you of or say to you? If you are able, put your ear against the plant's stem, trunk, leaf, or flower. Close your eyes and listen deeply.

7. Pay attention to how your body feels. It may be that your body feels different when you are with the plant. Perhaps you experience physical sensations of some kind? If so, where in your body do you feel these sensations? How does your body respond to the plant? What can your body tell you?

8. Take your awareness deep inside yourself and become aware of your emotions. How are you feeling emotionally? Many times a plant will communicate through human emotions. Have your feelings changed since being with the plant?

9. Is there a word or phrase that comes to mind that sums up your sense of this plant? If so, remember this word, as it can be a helpful reminder of your experience and a shortcut to revisiting the plant.

10. Spend time with the plant, simply being. Let go of expectations and just enjoy the company of this amazing plant. Ask the plant to come to the empty space inside of you. Allow your mind to be a blank screen, and receive whatever is given. If your mind wanders, just allow thoughts to ripple away, and return yourself to your intention to connect with the plant. You might like to sing to the plant or play a musical instrument. If you are a visual type of person, you may see images of the plant spirit. This is likely to come in a form that has meaning for you personally. As humans,

we often project human characteristics onto nature spirits and all of this is valuable, although it does not necessarily mean the plant spirits actually look as we see them. It may be that you have a conversation with the plant and can ask many questions. On the other hand, you might receive healing from the plant and you may or may not have any memory of this afterward. Anything can happen, and you can trust that whatever occurs is the perfect experience for you; nothing is right or wrong. There is no value in making judgments or comparisons. Accept whatever is given, and know that every day is different and everyone perceives differently. Honor your own experience.

11. Finally, when the time comes to return, give your thanks to the plant and leave a gift. This gift can be anything that is natural and nontoxic for the plant, the land, or local animals. It is a gift from your heart. I often use blessing herbs, such as lavender or rose petals, small stones or crystals, flower essences, a song, or a simple kiss.

Essentially, you are training yourself to tune in with the plant, to be on the same frequency. This is natural and easy. For most humans it takes practice simply because we have to undo the false conditioning that our minds have received since childhood. Listen to your heart, and trust your first impressions. You are making a new friend; get to know this being in every way possible. Let it become a true relationship of intimacy.

## 🌿 A NATIVE AMERICAN METHOD FOR CONNECTING WITH PLANTS

Another beautiful way of connecting with plants is inspired by Native American mystic Joseph Rael, also known as Beautiful Painted Arrow, a mixed Southern Ute and Picuris Pueblo Indian.*

1. Touch the plant and close your eyes as you focus on feeling the plant with your fingertips. Go deeper and deeper as you merge through touch— stroking, patting, caressing.

2. As you do this, listen carefully for the sound of the plant. Keep listening

---

*See www.josephrael.org.

closely until you pick up the vibration. You may see images with your inner eye. You may receive an inner smell or taste. You can make a song from the vibration. Just let it come. Sing to the plant and with the plant.

3. Now, let your body move with this song. Dance to it. Let the vibration move throughout your body. Keep going until you feel you have merged with the sound and with the plant.

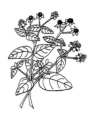

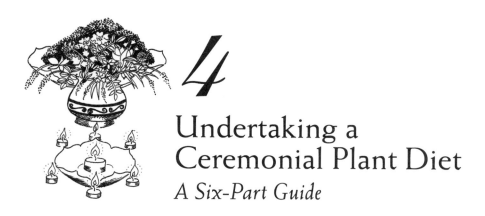

# 4

# Undertaking a Ceremonial Plant Diet
*A Six-Part Guide*

*Sacred Ones of the Plant World,*
*I align my intent with the intent of Grandmother Earth and all*
*her Worlds,*
*I open my heart in gratitude,*
*I open my heart in awe and wonder,*
*May I walk in Beauty this day and all days,*
*May I be guided in the making of an elixir of Beauty*
*That honors the plants and expresses your Dream.*
*And may this elixir bring Blessings to the plants and to all the*
*Worlds of the Grandmother.*

The basic steps involved in undertaking a ceremonial plant diet include the following:

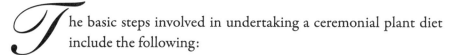 Setting a sacred intention for your plant diet
 Choosing a plant to diet
 Harvesting the plant and preparing the elixir
 Spiritual and physical preparation for the plant diet

❧ Carrying out the diet

❧ Integration

## STEP 1: SETTING A SACRED INTENT

The first crucial step is to set a strong and clear intention. The prime intent is to honor the plants and their gifts and to develop a diet that will offer the very best possible to all those involved, in service of the highest good of all.

Effectively, the diet begins as soon as the intent has been set. As maker of the elixir, it may be that you first set the intention to do a plant diet and then decide which plant to use. These two steps often occur simultaneously, sometimes well in advance of the physical making.

## STEP 2: DECIDING WHICH PLANT TO DIET

I have to admit that as a passionate plant enthusiast I would like to diet with just about every species I can think of, but that isn't practical so I have to be selective. Usually the initial idea or message comes in a flash and then develops over time. I perceive it as a calling from the plants. I wait to see how the idea grows as I engage with the plants on the land. Typically, there are many more plants calling to be dieted than I can possibly accommodate, so I engage in a co-creative process to determine which plants to work with. Essentially I am asking Spirit to guide me to choose the best plant for the good of all. Sometimes the call from a plant is so strong that it really feels like a hammer on the head!

Recently, we dieted here with Borage. This decision was reached during a conversation with one of the group who intended to come. It was high summer and many plants were coming forward to be dieted at Lughnasadh, the harvest festival. Several were tempting me. During my conversation with this woman, I realized that she needed some specific help, and I simply asked silently to know the next plant we should diet. My entire mind was instantly filled with Borage flowers. Our subsequent Borage plant diet turned out to be perfect both for her needs and for what the whole group needed at that time.

Once the plant is chosen, I am dreaming with that plant in both the waking and sleeping dream, receiving guidance, gathering information and insights, and establishing a deeper relationship. Where it is appropriate, I like to use several different parts of the plant in an elixir. For instance, with Dog Rose I could use both the flowers and the rosehips, as well as small amounts of root, stem, and leaf. In these instances, the making of the elixir can take many months because different parts need to be harvested at different times of year. As with everything in Nature, we need to be patient and allow the medicine to evolve in its own right timing.

For the rest of the participants, the diet begins once they commit to taking part. Initially the effects may be very subtle. These effects generally grow stronger as the time of the diet draws closer.

## STEP 3: HARVESTING THE PLANT AND MAKING THE ELIXIR

For each plant diet I make a preparation called an elixir. This is a liquid extract of the plant to be dieted and is the sacrament to be ingested during the plant-diet ceremony. The timing and specific method of making an elixir is different for each diet, depending on how I am guided. To develop the plant diets I rely on inner guidance (this being guidance that sometimes directs me to outer sources of information like textbooks, for example). I perceive this guidance as coming from the plants themselves, together with my higher self, my intuition, and assistance from other nonphysical beings—sometimes called nature spirits, devas, angels, and ancestors. This guidance is combined with my own existing body of plant knowledge. Occasionally I use additional techniques, such as dowsing or muscle testing, to verify what I am doing. The individual methods used for the diets described in this book are outlined in the separate plant chapters. My intention is to be guided to make an elixir that will bring through all the qualities that the plant wants to offer humans at this time, and that are right for all who are taking part. In other words, as in the Beauty Way tradition, I intend to make an elixir of beauty, and this is for the highest good of all and according to the free will of all. This last statement is designed to ensure that nothing in the making or ingestion of the elixir goes against anyone's free will. Put another way, it means that no being, including invisible beings, is being manipulated in any way. Other personal or collective intents may be added to this.

Harvesting the plant and making the elixir are both done in ceremony. These ceremonies may be as simple or as complex as you choose. Either way it means there is a conscious honoring of Spirit and a bringing together of physical and nonphysical realms. Usually I am doing this as a lone human, although I am regularly accompanied by animals such as my dogs or cats. It is not necessary to follow a particular spiritual tradition. Be authentic. Be respectful. Follow your heart. If you don't have experience communicating with plants, it will first be helpful to practice the exercises in the previous chapter, "Connecting with the Spirit of Plants."

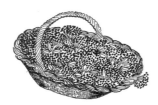

## Part 1: Harvesting

Harvesting for the elixir involves spending time with the plants, listening and watching, being appreciative, asking for permission, and paying attention so that you know the correct time and the correct parts to harvest. The correct time to harvest will in part be determined by the time of year and the growth and development of the plant (for example, you can't harvest Hawthorn berries in springtime!). If you are not familiar with plant identification, you will need a field guide to be sure you have the correct plants. Furthermore, if you are unfamiliar with the medicinal use of plants, you will need a good medicinal herbal to know what parts of the plant can be used and when best to pick them. Many plants will immediately come forward and offer themselves. On the other hand, and especially if you do not already have a close relationship with the plant you want to harvest, you may find that a plant needs to be carefully courted before you can pick it. It may even be that your chosen plant requires hunting, and this may be part of a warrior quest that assists your own personal development.

If you happen to have chosen a poisonous plant then great care will be needed in the making of the elixir and the design of the ceremony. DO NOT INGEST TOXIC PLANTS unless you really know the maximum safe dosage. This is not an area to be approached lightly. You can easily kill yourself by ingesting wild plants. However, some of the poisonous plants offer potent initiations. If one of these is calling you strongly, you could try doing a different kind of plant diet. For instance, you could take the flower essence, inhale the scent or essential oil, or if appropriate, soak in a gentle foot or hand bath. You need to thoroughly research and know the plant in advance. Ideally, find someone with experience who can advise you. Remember that toxic plants tend to have powerful personalities and must always be treated with the utmost respect.

Harvesting will also be determined by weather conditions, and you may want to consider planetary aspects. Several helpful books on these topics are listed in the bibliography at the end of this book. For general purposes, it is often best to pick herbs on a sunny day after the dew has dried. However, for ceremonial purposes, you may want to harvest under the light of the full moon or at some other specific time. Ask for guidance from Spirit in advance, stay attentive for signs, and follow your intuition and common sense. I often sing or play music to the plants while I'm harvesting, thanking them and celebrating their beauty and other attributes. Frequently a song will come while I'm out on the land with the plants. This may be a song for singing at the initiation ceremony or simply one to sing to the plants in the moment and/or later during the making of the elixir. I do my best to be fully present and to pay attention to everything that is going on around me, since I have learned that whatever happens during these times has significance for the entire plant diet.

My personal approach is to ask the plants to show me which of them (and which parts) would like to be picked. Who wants to be part of this elixir? I first explain what I am doing and ask if they are happy with that. If I am picking away from home, I always introduce myself first. It may be that you will notice one or more Grandfather or Grandmother plants.

These are often larger and more imposing than those of the same variety around them. They are like the head of the family. Don't pick these unless you are certain it is being asked for.

Naturally, if you are harvesting in the wild, it must be done responsibly. Only ever take a small proportion of what is growing in any one area. Do not harvest from beside a busy road or where toxic spraying has taken place. Be sure to know your plants and do not pick endangered species. You may want to avoid picking the first plant you see of any particular species. In the Mohawk tradition, it is taught that the first plant you see should be the one you offer thanks to because this plant is still with us, performing its duty, and you wish it to continue. You are advised to walk past the first plant and look for another one, this being the one to pick. You do not pick the first one because, for all you know, it may be the last one existing in the world.

Sometimes additional helper plants are called for in an elixir. This may be a plant or a group of plants that have traditionally been used to complement the primary plant. Alternatively, it may be a seemingly unrelated plant that simply calls out to you. Be open to receiving this information from Spirit, and be sure you know how to use the plant safely.

**Giving Offerings:** This important topic deserves a special mention. An offering is a gift of energy that comes from the heart, and giving offerings is an important way to give thanks and blessings when harvesting plants. Fresh blossoms, a pinch of dried herbs, or a small crystal or stone can all make effective offerings. Generally I carry an offering pot or offering bag whenever I am out on the land. This is a small jar or fabric bag that fits easily into a pocket and contains items such as dried rose petals or buds, small crystals, dried lavender, or cornmeal. A pinch of herbs or a small crystal can be offered to a plant as the need arises. Similarly, you could leave a small home-baked cake or similar item. Handmade goods have particular value because you have put something of yourself into them. Offerings must be nontoxic to the environment and to the other creatures around. Chocolate should be avoided because it is toxic to most animals due to its theobromine content. A small pinch of Tobacco is a traditional Native American blessing or Tobacco flower essence can be given. Tobacco is a sacred power plant with many ceremonial uses. For instance, to the Kicka-poo Nation, the sharing of Tobacco or its smoke deepens relationships between beings and extends communication. Flower essences make excellent offerings, as can sprinklings of herbal infusions or decoctions. Milk can be a favorite offering for the faery folk or it can be mixed with honey to please the water spirits. Alcohol, such as a good quality whisky, can be poured as a libation at the feet of a plant, and incense can be burned with the smoke providing a sweet-smelling gift. Candles can be lit (being careful to clear them away later) and for trees it is a Celtic tradition to tie pieces of cloth to their branches. This is akin to the Native American tradition of making prayer ties where prayers are offered with each tie. Plants are particularly fond of music and song. I often sing to the plants or play my small finger piano, drum, or harp. You can offer beautiful words of praise and adoration, recite poetry, or do vocal toning. You can also caress the plant, connecting from the heart and letting loving energies flow through your hands or on your breath as a kiss. The important thing is that any offering authentically comes from the heart.

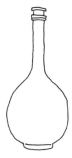

## *Part 2: Making the Elixir*

An elixir can be as plain as a simple infusion of the plant or it may be complex, as in a combination of more than one extract from the same plant species. For example, dieting with Meadowsweet could simply involve making a tea from leaves and flower buds, harvested just before or during flowering. The fresh infusion would be taken in divided doses throughout the plant-diet ceremony. Alternatively, for a diet with Dog Rose you might like to include extracts of both the flowers and the berries (or hips), which by necessity would be harvested at different times of the year. These extracts would therefore need preserving and would then be combined to make the elixir just prior to the plant diet. In the later chapters for each plant included, I describe two different methods I have used for making their elixirs. For the diets I have developed, you will notice that the actual processes of harvesting and making elixirs can vary widely, even for the same plant when it is dieted more than once.

Chapter 5, "Herbal Basics," provides easy instructions for making standard herbal preparations, which can be used to make plant elixirs. If you are new to making plant extracts you could start simply with an herbal tea. I include instructions for other forms of extracts, which you may be inspired to try out if you want to develop more complex elixirs. This is an opportunity to be creative! Whatever you choose to do, any extract must be prepared in a sacred manner with an attitude of respect and honoring for the plant. Typically, just prior to the diet, there is a final ceremonial mixing and blessing. This involves prayer and contemplation or meditation. It commonly includes activities such as singing, playing instruments or recorded music, blowing in prayers with smoke (or breath), and the channeling of energies through the hands or other means. Tobacco is a strong and sacred ally for me and assists in the making of elixirs. It is not required for use unless you have a personal relationship with it and feel genuinely guided to incorporate it.

## STEP 4: PREPARING YOURSELF FOR A PLANT DIET

A plant diet may be undertaken alone or in a group. Working in a group can enhance and magnify the effects, as well as provide a source of human support. On the other hand, it may be that you are seeking time alone with your plant of choice and this can be equally rewarding.

The spirit of the plant and the intent of the initiate are paramount. If you have been making the elixir then you will have already set your intention, but you may want to refine it still further as the main ceremony approaches. If this is to be a group ceremony, then it is helpful for all participants to start forming their intentions as early as possible. In general, the stronger your intent, the more potent the effects of the diet will be.

Ask yourself, why am I doing this diet? What are my deepest intentions? On a certain level, the ceremony begins for each person from the moment he or she commits to participate.

You will need to decide how long your diet will last. This is entirely up to you. Starting out, I would suggest around two days. Most of the ceremonies described in this book took place over the course of two or three days. Some plant diets can last for weeks or months. If you have a strong calling, you might want to set a longer diet up for yourself. It will certainly change your life.

Personal preparation includes a period of physical purification. This helps you to be clearer and more receptive to the plant. Generally we prepare our bodies for at least three days in advance. Typically this involves excluding meat and dairy products, refined sugar, alcohol, strong spices, artificial additives, and coffee. Salt should be kept to a minimum, as well as soy or fermented products. In many traditions, participants in a plant diet are advised not to have sex in the days beforehand (as well as during and afterward, while they integrate the experience). This can be viewed as an additional way of keeping your energy clear and contained. I find that this practice aids the connection with the plant (particularly with some who may be more demanding than others). However, there are no rigid taboos. It is entirely between you and the plant; therefore, it is your own personal decision. Simply ask the plant! With nonpsychoactive plants, the purpose of preparatory purification is entirely to enhance the effects of the diet. You will be more receptive and the plant will have an easier way into your body. Personal safety is not an issue while eating particular foods to prepare for a diet with nonpsychoactive plants. This is unlike diets with certain psychoactive plants,* which may possibly be dangerous if taken in conjunction with particular foods. One physical benefit of preparing your body in this way is that withdrawal effects from physical addictions like coffee or sugar are likely to have passed by the time of commencing the diet. On this note, it may sometimes be helpful to avoid additional substances such as wheat

---

*Ayahuasca, for instance, is a monoamine oxidase inhibitor (MAOI) and should not be taken alongside foods with high tyramine content, often found in aged and fermented foods.

in the preparatory stage. Interestingly, plant initiates here in Derrynagittah increasingly find that the plant to be dieted may start having a potent effect during these three preparatory days.

# STEP 5: CONDUCTING A PLANT DIET

## *Fasting*

During a plant diet, participants either fast completely or follow a specified restricted diet. Again, this helps us to be as clear and receptive as possible during the ceremony. In advance of the diet, I tune in to the plant and ask to know which foods and drinks will act in the most harmonious way with the elixir. These items are made available throughout the time of the diet. As with the preparatory diet, it is not that other foods will be unsafe, rather that people are likely to receive maximum benefit from the plant by adhering to the diet. Generally I find that most people aim to fast completely and rarely eat the specified foods. Some people choose to avoid all additional drinks including water. Each person is encouraged to be in his or her own self-authority, free to make personal decisions about food and drink consumption.

Fasting, in and of itself, is possibly the most ancient of all self-healing techniques and can bring enormous physical benefits. It speeds up the elimination of metabolic waste and has a purifying effect on the body. In many traditions, fasting is encouraged as a spiritual discipline to help a person feel more connected to Spirit. It allows us to review our relationship with food and it can bring all kinds of emotional issues to the surface. In the context of a plant diet, fasting purifies us, it helps us to be receptive to the plant, and it also facilitates healing by making our issues more accessible.

Anyone who needs to eat or drink for medical reasons should, of course, do so. Any eating should be done discreetly so as not to disturb others. The dietary restrictions are not about denial of our needs but rather the letting go of self-imposed limitations that may block us from our highest potential. The intention is for each person to come to the ceremony in a way that honors the sacred and his or her own process, while being as open as possible to the plant on all levels.

## Establishing Sacred Space

Before any ceremony is performed, it is essential to call on the guardian spirits of the place where it will be held. If the guardian spirits do not want a ceremony to take place, they may easily disrupt it in some way, obvious or otherwise. Simply greet the guardians and ask permission for your ceremony to take place. A simple statement like the one below will suffice:

> *Hail, Guardians of this Sacred Place! I come as _____ (your name), in peace and with respect, asking for permission to do a plant-diet ceremony here this weekend. I ask you to accept my/our presence.*

You must check inside yourself for the response, doing your best to discern between what may be your own internal hopes and fears and a genuine energetic response from Spirit. Answers can come in many ways. For instance the sun may suddenly emerge from behind a cloud, a bird may sing, or you may simply feel warm and happy.

A plant initiation ceremony is a sacred event needing a clear and focused atmosphere, as free as possible from the distractions of daily life. Before starting, you need to establish sacred space by consecrating the area. Sacred space requires an environment that is clear, clean, and safe. Set your intention to create this within yourself as well. Choose your space with care. At Derrynagittah we work in a ten-sided sound temple that is dedicated to sacred ceremony. Whether you are in a dedicated temple, your own home sitting room, or a quiet place in Nature, the space needs to be a beautiful, safe container with well-defined boundaries where you will not be disturbed. The ceremonial area needs to be physically clean. This sounds obvious but it's an important consideration! Next, the area and all your working tools must be smudged, meaning they are to be cleansed with sacred smoke. I usually use Sage or a special blend of herbs. This is like the practice of burning incense in church. Sage, or other herbs and resins, is burned to create smoke that cleanses the space and your items. In many traditions, smoke is seen to inhabit both the visible physical world and the invisible spirit world because it has no substance. I also use vibrational essence sprays to bring additional qualities to the space.* These can be used for purification as well as for bringing protection and blessings. Furthermore, if you prefer not to use smoke, essence sprays can provide an effective alternative.

An altar should be set up in advance, preferably in the center of the space. This is a doorway between the human world and the world of Spirit. It provides a focal point for connecting with and honoring the Divine. An altar can be as simple as a candle and flowers, or it may be a complex design of many sacred objects. You can use a small table or chest, or you could place a beautiful cloth on the floor. Consider the intention of the altar. What is its sacred purpose? For a plant initiation, your altar will celebrate and connect with the plant being dieted (see color plate 3). Have this purpose clear in your mind, and make a simple statement dedicating your altar to its sacred objective. Every item placed on the altar should be meaningful to you, and each item should hold a resonance, meaning that it is vital with power and energy. Think of the difference between a vibrant, freshly picked plant and a withered, dried-up specimen. Generally, a plant initiation altar is likely to be adorned with the plant being dieted as well as with the bottles of plant elixir ready for drinking. The plant in question could be represented by fresh or dried plant material, or by photographs or other art work. My altars usually contain an object to represent each of the four elements. For instance, I might use incense or a feather for Air in the East; a candle for Fire in the South; a goblet of water, mead, or the plant elixir for Water in the West; and a dish of earth or a rock for Earth in the North. Alternatively, you could use specific plants or crystals appropriate to each of the elements. If the ceremony is also celebrating a particular Fire Festival then this can be similarly reflected in the altar.

You may want to bathe or shower before starting the ceremony. You are aiming to come to meet this plant in as pristine a state as possible, of

---

*See "Resources" on page 288 for details of vibrational essence sprays.

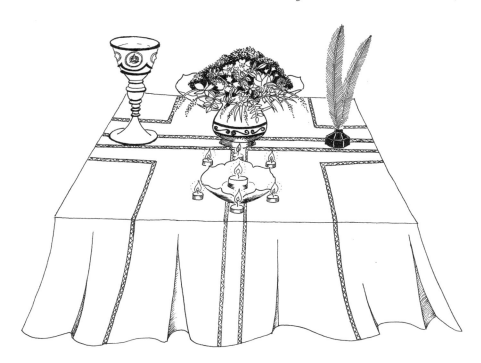

*An altar set up to honor the four elements*

body, mind, and spirit. You also want to present yourself to Spirit in a beautiful and honoring way. Therefore you might choose to wear clothes that are reserved for sacred ceremony or at least wear something that feels like you have made an effort! Wristwatches should be removed in advance, as their vibrations can be disruptive. All participants should be smudged when they arrive. This cleanses their energy field and is a way to clear out mental and emotional debris and to become psychologically prepared for a shift in consciousness.

In our plant initiations, participants pick a tarot card on arrival. This gives them guidance on the energies they are working with and the kind of challenges and gifts they may personally encounter with this plant. In a group context, each card represents an aspect of the group since we are all connected. You can use any of the many divination packs that are widely available.

## *Focused Intent*

Sitting with our tarot cards, we quiet our minds and focus on our intent. By quieting the mind we create an empty space that can be filled. Part of our intention is to surrender to the plant. We align our intents with Spirit and do our best to let go of our ego's expectations and control and simply let the plant take over. People set their own personal intents. It is appropriate to set an intention for whatever will nourish you in your life. That way the energy can flow through you to others. Don't worry that you are being "selfish." Together with your personal intent, you set an intention for your community, the local environment, the entire planet, and beyond. I always intend that the ceremony send blessings to the plant being dieted and to all the worlds of Grandmother Earth.

Be aware that these initiations can take us to very deep places where hidden aspects of ourselves can unexpectedly emerge for integration, healing, or review. During ceremony we may contact what psychoanalyst C. G. Jung called the shadow self, aspects of ourselves that we have shunned or disowned and that we may be unaware of in ordinary life. This unowned shadow material can contaminate our inner life as well as our actions in the world. Acknowledging our shadow is an enormously helpful part of our own development. During a plant initiation we need to be mindful that we do not inadvertently, or otherwise, send unhelpful energies to others, that we don't dump our "stuff" on anyone else or make them responsible for our feelings. Therefore, at the start of ceremony we also intend that we will not pass on anything harmful to any other being. The traditional Wiccan creed "And it harm none" is always appropriate.

## *Invocation*

With our intentions clear, we center ourselves by taking our consciousness inside to feel the depth of our being. One way to help still the mind is to take slow, deep breaths. We spend time focusing on our physical heart and feeling gratitude. Aware of our own sacred nature and feeling our connection to the Earth beneath our feet and the Sky above us, it is now time to sanctify the space by invoking God, Goddess, the

Gods, Holy Spirit, Great Spirit, or whatever is your own understanding of Spirit. You may want to construct a ceremonial circle to work within—creating a protected, sacred space symbolic of the whole world, a microcosm of the macrocosm. You are invoking sacred presence, asking for blessings and protection, respectfully welcoming the incoming energies, and stating your intentions to Spirit. There is no fixed way to do this, although there are traditionally proven ways you can usefully follow, paths that have been forged by others that can guide and protect your way. Equally, you can be open to new ways of being in ceremony. After all, a living spirituality needs to grow and change and ceremony is ultimately a vehicle for mystery. Invoke whatever feels appropriate to the time and place and people involved. Speak from the heart and make your invocations with a sense of presence and connection.

Below is a simple method of invocation you can use at plant-diet ceremonies. This can be used as a model and modified according to your own belief system and preferences. This model calls to the four elements that make up life: Air, Fire, Water, and Earth. Each of these is presided over by elemental spirits or guardians and each one holds different representational qualities. Air represents the mind; Fire the spark of life, the vital energy; Water the emotions; Earth the physical body. Each element is also associated with a particular direction. In the Celtic tradition Air is associated with the East, Fire with the South, Water with the West, and Earth with the North. Next, call to the "As above" and the "So below". "As above, so below" is a maxim referring to the unity of all things. What is above us reflects below, just as what is inside of us reflects what is outside. Above us is the celestial realm, including angels, archangels, sun, moon, stars, planets, and the rest of the Cosmos. Below is the deep, primal land of the ancestors and the spirits of minerals, plants, and animals. This is also the land of the faery folk and the Shining Ones, the Tuatha dé Danaan. Ultimately, all the realms merge as one great Circle. Now take your attention to the Center. This is the center of all existence and the place of Great Mystery, the Spirit within all of life. Address Spirit and all who have gathered from the invisible world, stating your intentions for ceremony.

## 🌿 CALLING TO THE DIRECTIONS

Be clear with yourself (or the group, if you are working with one) that you are creating sacred space. As you call to each direction, see, sense, or feel the energy as strongly as you are able.

### East

Walk to the East direction.

Facing the East, raise your hands, palms facing forward, and say:

*"Guardians of the East, elemental power of Air, be present, guard, and protect this circle. Hail and welcome!"*

Visualize, sense, or feel the presence of Air.

See rushing winds. Hear birdsong. Feel the breath of life, inspiration.

### South

Walking around the Circle clockwise, go to the South direction.

Facing the South, raise your hands, palms facing forward, and say:

*"Guardians of the South, elemental power of Fire, be present, guard, and protect this circle. Hail and welcome!"*

Visualize, sense, or feel the presence of Fire.

See flames, the gold, orange, red of the noonday sun. Feel heat, the vitality of Fire, energy, passion, and creativity.

### West

Walk to the West direction.

Facing the West, raise your hands, palms facing forward, and say:

*"Guardians of the West, elemental power of Water, be present, guard, and protect this circle. Hail and welcome!"*

Visualize, sense, or feel the presence of Water.

See waves, water, rivers, and lakes. See the color blue. Feel flow, imagination, healing, intuition, and enchantment.

### North

Walk to the North direction.

Facing the North, raise your hands, palms facing forward, and say:

*"Guardians of the North, elemental power of Earth, be present, guard, and protect this circle. Hail and welcome!"*

Visualize, sense, or feel the presence of Earth.

See dark soil, mountains, cliffs, rolling hills, and valleys. Feel groundedness and stability, nurture and abundance.

### Above

Walk to the Center.

Facing the altar, lift your arms to the Sky, and say:

*"I call Above, to you of the stars and planets, angels and celestial beings, all who come in Peace. Hail and welcome!"*

Visualize, sense, or feel the presence of all from Above.

Envision stars, planets, and outer space. Feel the presence of celestial beings.

### Below

Lower your arms to the Earth, and say:

*"I call Below, to you, luminous beings of inner Earth, all who come in Peace. I call to the ancestors, minerals, plants, and animals. I call to you _____ (plant name), you who I/we will diet with over the next days. Thank you for your presence. Hail and welcome!"*

Visualize, sense, or feel the presence of all from Below.

See the vibrant, primal landscape and be aware of the presence of your ancestors and allies. Feel the strong presence of the plant you are about to diet with.

### Center

Bring your hands back to your heart, saying:

*"I call to Spirit in the Center! Great Spirit, Great Mystery, the Void, the All, and the Everything: Come, I/we honor your presence."*

Feel the presence of Spirit alive within every cell of your body and within everything around you.

### Speak Your Intentions

Now, state your intentions:

*"Sacred and Holy Ones, I/we come in Peace and with pure intent.*

*I/We come today to diet with the sacred _____ (plant name).*

Clearly speak your intentions for the initiation.

*"Let this be a ceremony of beauty that honors _____ (plant name) and brings*

blessings to all of its kind. Let this ceremony bring blessings to all the worlds of Grandmother Earth, for the highest good of all and according to the free will of all."

You may want to invite participants to state their intentions out loud to Spirit. If you are working with a group this can be done going clockwise around the circle, each person being encouraged to speak simply and from the heart, finishing with "Blessed Be," "Amen," "Aho," or whatever is appropriate for them.

### Create the Container

Still standing at the center, focus your gaze on the East of the circle, saying:

*"May this circle be protected."*

Visualize a blue flame arising in the East and sweeping around the circle clockwise forming a protective ring of blue Fire around the outside of your ceremonial space. Feel and know that all within the circle are held in safety and protection. This provides a safe sanctuary for the initiates while allowing them to come and go from the circle as they choose. Now, state aloud:

*"Blessed Be!"*

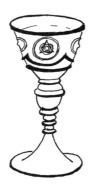

## Ingesting the Elixir

With sacred space created and Spirit invoked, you are now ready to start drinking the elixir. This is ingested at regular intervals, for us at Derrynagittah usually over a period of two to three days. The first serving is given to Grandmother Earth as an offering and I then pour drinks for the participants. During the ceremony I will dispense the elixir as appropriate, perhaps six to eight times. Generally this will be an equal amount for each person but the quantity given may vary depending on the recipient. For instance, if someone is having a very strong response it may (or may not) be best for them to receive only a small dose or to even miss a few doses. I seek guidance from Spirit, combined with common sense, and experience. One way to get reinforcement from Spirit is to tap the cup against the bottle of elixir while whispering the person's name and wait for an internal or external indication. Pregnancy is a special case. I would not recommend that you give an elixir to a pregnant or breast-feeding woman unless you have specialist knowledge of herbal medicine in pregnancy. Without ingesting the elixir, a pregnant or breast-feeding woman can still attend the ceremony in order to meditate and spend time with the plant. If appropriate, the elixir can be applied via the skin.

As already stated, many of the plant diets at Derrynagittah are timed to coincide with the Fire Festivals. By celebrating these festivals we are tuning in to the cycles of Nature and this facilitates access to the plant world. Furthermore, these are times when powerful energies affect the planet and add potency to any plant initiation. Diets may of course be carried out at any time and may be timed with lunar or other planetary events or with your own health requirements. For instance, a Hawthorn initiation might be helpful for someone with high blood pressure whereas a Nettle diet can be beneficial for a person with a skin complaint like eczema. Massive healing shifts can take place at these initiations.

## Dreaming with the Plant

For the duration of the ceremony, we engage in various activities that help us to deepen our relationship with the plant; to get to know it better, to bond, to blend, and if we can, to merge. We call this dreaming with the plant. We enter into alternate reality and connect with the plant's consciousness. This can be while awake or sleeping. Specific activities are determined by many factors, including the plant itself, the people present, and the timing of the diet. We surrender to Spirit and enter into the unknown. As the leader of the group, I am responsible for holding a place of safety for others and for being both a guide and an anchor. At times it may be helpful to remind a person to return to his or her heart center, to relax, breathe deeply, and surrender to the plant.

Activities frequently include making inner journeys with the plant. We travel using drum, rattle, silence, other instruments, voice, or prerecorded sound. We spend time with the plant in Nature, connecting and giving blessings as a group or individually. We invite the plant into our bodies, becoming conscious of how it moves through our energy centers and tissues. Participants may be anointed with the plant or take plant baths. We may express the plant through creative activities such as mask making, or working with clay, poetry, song, chanting, toning, dancing, or other movement. We may invite the plant to speak through us or listen to its stories in myth and folklore. We might sit in meditation with its picture or work with it in the labyrinth or the medicine wheel. We frequently incorporate GreenBreath, a method of joining with a plant through music and breath (see "Resources" on page 288 for further information), and I might discuss the plant's medicinal actions. With a plant biofeedback device, I sometimes incorporate the songs of the plants. The possibilities are endless.

Throughout the period of the plant diet we sleep in the ceremonial space and record our experiences and dreams. During these ceremonies, we open ourselves to powerful, transformative energies that exist in the ceremonial space. On the last day, we sit together and share what has been revealed through our experiences. We are present for each other with active listening, mainly keeping a respectful silence without interpretation or discussion, although sometimes it is helpful for me to ask questions. This sharing is a significant part of the diet and can afford profound insights and healing, both for the individual and the collective. At the end of the ceremony it is vital that we give thanks and release all the beings who have helped us, intending that the blessings given will "grow corn" in our lives, meaning that they will be of practical value in the world, giving nourishment and facilitating authentic beneficial change. We offer prayers that blessings will radiate out to our communities and to all of life. After giving our thanks, a traditional way to release our spirit helpers and close the ceremony is to state "Hail and Farewell!" We finish with a celebratory feast. It is important that everyone has some food and drink prior to leaving in order to be grounded before venturing back into the outside world.

Appendix 2, "Summary Steps for Performing a Ceremonial Plant Diet," provides a simplified format for carrying out your own initiations. In addition, specially recorded audio tracks for use at your plant diets can be downloaded from the Inner Traditions • Bear & Company website at audio .innertraditions.com/saplin. See appendix 4, "How to Use the Plant Initiation Audio Tracks." Allow yourself to be inspired and guided by the plants!

## STEP 6: INTEGRATION

After the diet we may continue working with the plant by taking its flower essence, using an essence spray, or taking a low dose of the elixir for the following two to three weeks. This can help to stabilize and integrate the experience.

It is important to remember that you have taken part in what can be a very powerful ceremony and that given appropriate conditions, the plant may continue working in your body for some time afterward. Furthermore, you may have undergone a major transformation within yourself, and this needs time to integrate. I encourage people to be gentle with themselves, especially over the first few days following the diet. You may feel vulnerable and very different. This is normal. Often, participants will have received a new healing template, and this needs time to fully anchor. After the ceremony, I suggest that participants keep a seventy-two-hour discipline during which time, unless it is essential, they do not discuss what happened with anyone else, particularly anyone who was not present at the initiation. After this time, it is still important that you be careful whom you choose to share information with, hopefully only sharing with those who are supportive and nonjudgmental. These practices will help you to hold on to what has been received. If possible, go for walks in Nature, take time to listen to your favorite music, or do physical exercise that you enjoy. Do not put yourself under pressure or stresses. Try to ensure that you have as light a schedule as possible and give yourself time to integrate and absorb what you have experienced. Avoid getting into arguments. Choose light meals and avoid pork for about two to three days, as its protein is very dense. Some participants choose to continue with the preparatory diet for the following two to three weeks. Remember that your inner healer has received everything it needs, and this will continue to unfold in perfect timing. The diets may be gentle or intense. Either way, they can have a lasting effect, though the effects may not always be evident until later.

## Developing an Ongoing Relationship with the Plant

When a person attends a plant initiation, it is likely that the plant has called to him or her on the inner planes. This suggests that the plant can help with something in his or her life, whether personal or for the wider collective. As well as the time spent in ceremony, the plant may also be offering a longer-term relationship and very often, if the initiate is not already working with the plant, it comes forward as an ally. This is perhaps for a short while or perhaps for a lifetime. It may well be the start of a long and beautiful relationship! Sometimes the spirit of the plant enters the initiate and merges with his or her body. If this happens you receive strength and blessings from the plant and, through transmission, you can share these gifts with others. When a plant is particularly determined to stay with you, a strong ongoing relationship may happen automatically after a plant diet, and you will be well aware of the plant's presence in your life. Other times, if you want to maintain and develop your relationship with this potential ally, you must make efforts to sustain the relationship, just as you would with a human. For instance, you could grow the plant or regularly visit one of its kind in Nature, feeding it with your offerings (see information about offerings earlier in this chapter on pages 40–41). You could make an altar to the plant and tend it daily; you could study the plant in books, drink its tea, carry it on your person, or inhale the scent of its essential oil. There are countless ways to maintain and build your connection. If you ignore the plant, it may leave you. Talk to your new friend and ask what it would like, not only what it can do for you but also what you can do for it. This is a reciprocal relationship, a co-creation between the two of you, and many times a plant will have its own clear agenda. Pay attention to your dreams and chance encounters. Truly listen and be willing to act on what you hear. The request may be as simple as planting a seed or learning to take more time for yourself. You will not be expected to heal the entire planet. Generally we just have to start with the little bit that is close to us, our friends and loved ones, our community, and the earth beneath our feet. Each one of us can make a difference.

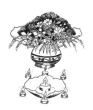

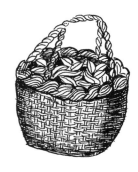

# 5

# Herbal Basics
## How to Make Standard Herbal Preparations

*I arise today with my heart full of gratitude.*
*I give thanks to you, Sacred Beings of the Plant World.*
*Thanks for your Beauty and Generosity,*
*Thanks for your Healing and Strength,*
*Thanks for your Inspiration and Guidance,*
*Thanks for your Love.*
*May I be guided by the power of Spirit to do your work.*
*Spirit, be in my hands, my heart, my mind!*
*Let thy will be my will.*
*Blessed Be!*

## HARVESTING HERBS

This chapter gives easy instructions for making standard herbal preparations, which can be used either singly or in combination to create a plant elixir. Read the harvesting guidelines in chapter 4 and if necessary refer to a good herbal book for detailed information specific to your chosen plant since individual recipes may vary (see the bibliography for recommendations).

## PREPARING HERBS

Most herbs can be used either fresh or dried. Here I am applying the definition of *herbs* as "useful plants," which for me covers every plant in existence! When harvesting leaves, stems, flowers, seeds, or berries there is no need to wash the plant material unless it is clearly covered in mud or other debris. It can be helpful to spread the parts out for a short while after picking in order for insects to escape. When using fresh aerial parts, they can be chopped and sometimes bruised just before use. This bruising can be done gently by hand, with the back of a spoon, a rolling pin, or a mortar and pestle, depending on how much you want to break down the cell walls. If you are unsure, refer to an herbal book for your specific plant and combine this knowledge with your own intuitive knowing. Roots will need to be scrubbed clean in water and can then be chopped into half-inch to one-inch pieces. For drying, aerial parts should not be washed and can be tied into small bunches and hung or spread out on trays. In either case, the place should be warm, dark, and airy. Similarly, chopped roots can be dried by spreading on a tray as outlined above or by placing the tray in an oven at its lowest setting for a few hours. After drying, the herb or root will feel brittle and dry to the touch. Dried herbs can be stored in airtight containers out of the sun, carefully labeled with name and date of harvest. Prepared extracts should also be labeled with name and date. Following are methods for making standard liquid preparations.

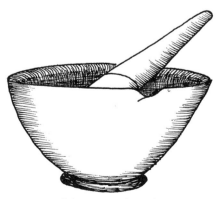

*Mortar and pestle*

# CHOOSING YOUR METHOD
## OF PREPARATION

Making an elixir often requires some forward planning—time of year and the availability of plant material being major factors that will influence your choice of method. If I know I want to diet a plant in winter, I usually have to harvest and prepare at least some of it in advance. Therefore, the component parts of an elixir may need to be prepared over a number of months and will need good keeping qualities. On the other hand, in summertime with an abundance of fresh plant material available, it is possible to be spontaneous and make elixirs for immediate ingestion. In addition, specific recipes may come to your attention at any time of year, and these can determine the makeup of your elixir. Ultimately, combined with practical knowledge and common sense, you need to follow your inspiration and inner guidance. The plant in question may be very clear that it wants to be prepared in a certain way.

A simple infusion or tea is one of the easiest and least expensive ways to prepare herbs. This is suitable for flowers, leaves, and other soft aerial parts of the plant. A decoction involves more vigorous extraction and is used for hard, woody material such as roots, bark, and berries. Both these methods are suitable if you are preparing an extract for nearly immediate use, as they have a short shelf life and will only keep for a maximum of three days in a cool place or refrigerator.

If you need more extended keeping properties, you can preserve infusions and decoctions by adding honey or sugar to turn them into syrups or by making herbal honeys. Alternatively, you can steep the plant in wine or beer or you can make your own beer or wine from the plant. You can also make an alcohol tincture. A tincture will keep for several years, is rapidly absorbed into the bloodstream, and provides a warming effect that helps to disperse the herbs in the body. I often make tinctures in advance and combine them with water extracts just before a plant diet.

If you prefer to avoid alcohol entirely, you can make a glycerite or vinegar, both of which last around two years. Infused oils are generally best kept for external use and make valuable anointing oils. Flower essences make a wonderful contribution to elixirs—you will generally need only a few drops for an entire elixir.

## Water Infusions

Pour 20 fl oz./500 ml of boiling water over 2 oz./60 g of fresh herb or 1 oz./30 g dried. The water should be just off the boil, since vigorously boiling water disperses valuable volatile oils in the steam. Cover tightly and let stand for ten to twenty minutes for a gentle infusion, or overnight for a stronger medicinal effect. Strain before use. Water infusions will generally keep for up to three days in a refrigerator.

## Water Decoctions

Place 2 oz./60 g of fresh plant material or 1 oz./30 g dried in a pan (NOT aluminum) with 30 fl. oz./750 ml of freshly drawn water. Bring to a boil and simmer for between twenty minutes and one hour, until the volume has reduced by one third to one half (i.e., reduce to 15–20 fl. oz.). Remove from heat and strain through muslin or other fine cloth in a strainer. Squeeze out all the liquid and discard the herbs (which make excellent compost). The decoction will keep for up to three days in a refrigerator.

## Tinctures

The term *tincture* is typically used to refer to an alcohol extract where the properties of the plant are extracted and preserved in a mixture of alcohol and water. This combination extracts more plant constituents than pure water alone. As long as the alcohol content is at least 20 percent, the tincture will last for many years. Any type of spirit may be used in a tincture, although vodka is the most popular for home use, since it has no taste of its own and does not flavor the herbs. On the other hand, you might want a particular flavor or quality provided by a specific type of spirit. Similarly, wine may be used but because of its lower alcohol content the resultant tincture will not be as long lasting as a spirit extract. Quality of ingredients is important, so be sure to buy the best alcohol you can afford.

Fill a jar with chopped fresh herbs. Cover with vodka or other spirits, close the jar, and leave in a dark place for two to six weeks, shaking occasionally. Strain through muslin or another fine cloth. Squeeze out all the liquid and discard the herbs. If using dried herbs, measure 1 part herbs to 5 parts diluted alcohol (for example, 20 g herbs to 100 ml liquid). The alcohol can be diluted in the proportion of 2 parts alcohol to 1 part water.

## Wines and Beers

Many herbs can be brewed into wines and beers and these can then be incorporated into elixirs. In addition, herbs can be decocted in wine or beer instead of water. They can also simply be added to wine or beer and left to infuse in the same way we make a tincture.

## Glycerites

A glycerite is the equivalent of an alcohol tincture using vegetable glycerin instead of alcohol. The herbs are extracted and preserved in glycerin, a sweet liquid derived from palm or other oil and available in most pharmacies. Glycerin provides a useful and soothing alternative to alcohol for tincture making but is less effective at extracting some plant constituents. A glycerite will only last for around two years.

When using fresh plant material, pour undiluted vegetable glycerin over the herbs, using the same method as for tinctures. In this case, however, the jar should be left in the sun or a warm place to infuse. If using dried herbs, mix 3 parts vegetable glycerin with 2 parts water.

## Vinegars

Vinegars are tinctures made with vinegar rather than alcohol. In general, vinegar is weaker at extracting plant constituents, but it is much less expensive and better tolerated by most people. Some plant constituents extract better in vinegar's acid medium. Vinegar is excellent for extracting minerals from herbs, it helps the body's acid/alkaline balance, and it assists in digestion. Cider vinegar is particularly beneficial for health, being antibacterial and antifungal and boosting the immune system.

The addition of honey to a vinegar tincture (called an oxymel) will cut the bite of the vinegar. Vinegar tinctures should be stored in a cool, dark place and will last around two years. Vinegars can be made by following the same directions as for alcohol tinctures, substituting vinegar for alcohol.

## *Herbal Honeys*

In addition to its preservative qualities, honey acts as a natural antibiotic. Local honey can also help prevent allergies like hay fever. Herbs can be directly infused in honey. Fill a jar with chopped, fresh herbs and pour honey over them. Close the jar and leave it in the sun or a warm place for two to six weeks before straining. If preferred, the herbal honey can be gently heated in a double boiler to speed up the process. The honey will keep indefinitely.

## *Syrups*

In a syrup, sugar or honey is used as a preservative. Syrups make ideal cough remedies, with honey being particularly soothing. The added sweetness can also make certain herbs more palatable. A simple syrup can be made from an infusion or a decoction. Heat 20 fl. oz./500 ml of a standard infusion or decoction in a pan. Add 20 fl. oz./500 g honey or sugar and stir constantly over gentle heat until dissolved. Allow the mixture to cool and pour into a clean dark glass bottle with a cork stopper.

## *Infused Oils*

Infused plant oils can be incorporated into elixirs if required. Alternatively, these oils can be used during plant diets for anointing or massage. The plant material should be infused in a good quality vegetable oil such as sunflower, olive, or almond and either left on a sunny windowsill or heated in a double boiler. These are known respectively as cold or hot infused oils. A cold infused oil is suitable for delicate flowers like St. John's Wort or Mullein, which would be damaged by heating.

Cold Infused Oils: Pack a glass jar tightly with the flower heads or petals and cover completely with oil. Put the lid on and leave on a sunny windowsill for two to three weeks. At the end of this time, strain the oil through muslin and store in a dark glass bottle. If fresh flowers and sunshine are still available, the infused oil can be made stronger by repeating the process using the same oil with new flowers.

Hot Infused Oils: The following method is suitable for most other plants. Gather the plant on a dry day and leave it to wilt for a few hours so that some of the water content has evaporated. Put half of the chopped plant material into a heatproof container, cover with extra virgin olive oil, and place in a double boiler or saucepan of water, ensuring that the container is covered so that water will not splash into the oil. Heat the water and simmer for three hours. Strain the oil (in this case do not press with a wooden spoon since you do not want to extract water). Then pour the oil back over the remaining half of the plant material and repeat the process for another three hours. This makes a double-strength oil. Strain and leave the oil to settle. Then carefully pour off the oil, separating it from any water and plant residue that has settled out on the bottom of the container. Leaving water or residue in the oil would cause it to go rancid. Infused oils will keep for one year.

## Plant/Flower Essences

Plant and flower essences carry the vibration of the plant and can be sensitively made by you or purchased commercially. There are numerous different methods of preparation, the most common being the sun method, originally popularized by English physician Dr. Edward Bach in the 1930s. Using this method, the plant material is placed in spring water in an open glass bowl and left to sit in the sunshine (typically during the morning as the sun rises in the sky toward noon) where the plant transmits its vibration to the water. This water is later strained and combined in equal parts with brandy to make a Mother tincture. Two drops of Mother tincture are added to 2 tablespoons (30 ml) of brandy to make a stock essence, which is then ready for use. Vibrational essences will keep indefinitely. A description of Dr. Bach's original methods can be found in several publications, including *The Bach Flower Remedies* by Nora Weeks and Victor Bullen (see bibliography).

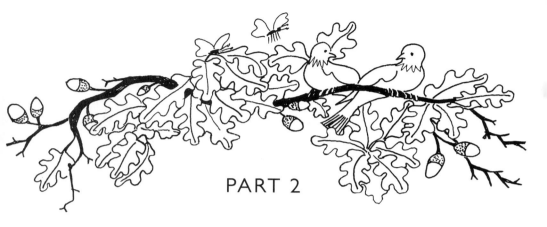

PART 2

# Entering the Dream of the Plants

### SACRED PLANT INITIATIONS
for the
EIGHT FIRE FESTIVALS

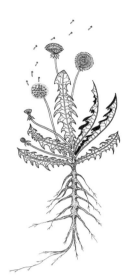

# Introduction to Part 2
## *The Wheel of the Year*

*T*he phrase *Wheel of the Year* describes Grandmother Earth's sacred cycle as She moves around Grandfather Sun. It charts the progression of the year's solar cycle and the eight Fire Festivals that have been celebrated since ancient times. As well as being important markers of the seasons, these festivals are astrological turning points. Each one highlights an important shift in the invisible forces acting on this planet. Observing these festivals is a significant aspect of social and spiritual life in Celtic lands as well as in many other places across the globe.

The Wheel of the Year is divided into eight subdivisions. Four fixed points known as the quarter points are crossed by four cross-quarter points. The quarter points are exact points determined by the position of the sun: the solstices when the days are longest and shortest, and the equinoxes when day and night are of equal length. Their exact times vary each year and can be found in a good almanac. Solstices and equinoxes were celebrated by our pre-Celtic ancestors. They constructed stone circles and monuments aligned to the position of the sun at these times. Christian festivals were superimposed upon these quarter points with Christmas and the birth of Jesus celebrated just after the Winter Solstice during the return of the Light. The cross-quarter points fall between the solstices and equinoxes. These are the great Celtic Fire Festivals of Samhain, Imbolc, Bealtaine, and Lughnasadh. Each of these can last for several days. The peak timing of their energy can vary depending on the position of the moon and other planetary bodies. For instance, the Celtic New Year is widely held to begin at the dark moon of Samhain (Late October/Early November), although opinions differ. The more you work consciously with the Wheel of the Year, the more it will enhance your awareness of Nature's presence within everything and of yourself as being a part of the whole.

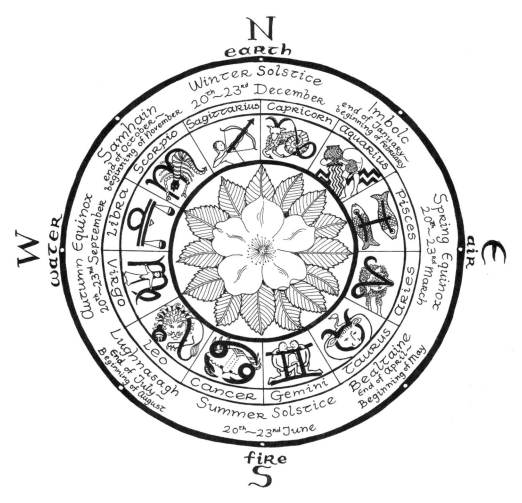

*The Wheel of the Year*

The plant initiations carried out at Derrynagittah are generally timed to coincide with these quarter and cross-quarter festivals. These times are powerful portals, giving access to potent energies from the Cosmos. By honoring and aligning with the turning of the Wheel of the Year, we venerate the Earth Herself, supporting Her transformation as well as our own. We also remember and honor the nature spirits during these festivals, aligning with them in order to establish a relationship based on mutual attention, respect, and cooperation. We affirm our awareness of being part of a Great Cosmic Cycle with the forces of Nature playing a fundamental role in our lives and evolution.

The following chapters will take you on a journey through the progression of Earth's sacred cycle, describing a particular plant in association with each of the eight Fire Festivals. These are not the only plants you could use. At Derrynagittah we have dieted with a range of plants for each festival, usually choosing those with traditional associations for the time of year in celebration. Information on plants associated with each festival can be found in appendix 3 as well as in some of the books listed in the bibliography. This book features one plant per festival. Drawing on my experience in herbal practice, each chapter gives a description of the plant, its folklore and history, and its use as an herbal medicine, a flower essence, and a spirit medicine. Bear in mind that each plant contains all of these overlapping qualities. The essence descriptions given are primarily for the essences that we have created at Derrynagittah. I outline the process of making plant elixirs and present our experiences from past ceremonies. The final chapter offers my conclusions. In addition to what you find here, please go to audio.innertraditions.com/saplin to find specially recorded audio tracks of guided meditations and music to help you carry out your own plant initiations.

Now, on to the adventure . . .

Led by Primrose, we join the Wheel at Bealtaine . . .

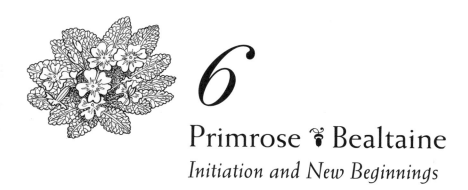

# 6

# Primrose ❦ Bealtaine
## Initiation and New Beginnings

rimrose comes as one of the first flowers of spring, offering light and hope after the darkness of winter. Ruled by Venus and considered female in gender, her bright yellow flowers surprise and delight us, lighting up the fields and bringing splashes of illumination to the woods and hedgerows (see color plate 4). She is associated with the element of Earth and with spring goddesses. The pale yellow-green of her petals carry a particular vibration, very different from Buttercup, Dandelion, or Lesser Celandine, which may all live close by. Sometimes alone and other times in large colonies covering an entire hillside, Primrose unlocks the spring and offers us a means to move forward. She is also known as the Key Flower, a gift from the gods and goddesses to show us the way to the hidden treasure inside ourselves and inside the Earth. Primrose offers us a key to go deep within and unlock riches that we may not have ever noticed. Change has come, light follows the darkness, and a shift has occurred. It is time to move toward the Light, time for initiation and rebirth into the freedom of our creative potential.

Associated with the growing life force of spring, Primrose has long been considered to have special powers. This is a traditional herb of Bealtaine (pronounced BEE-EL-TANA), bursting with bright, creative energy and initiating new beginnings. Primrose awakens both romantic love and

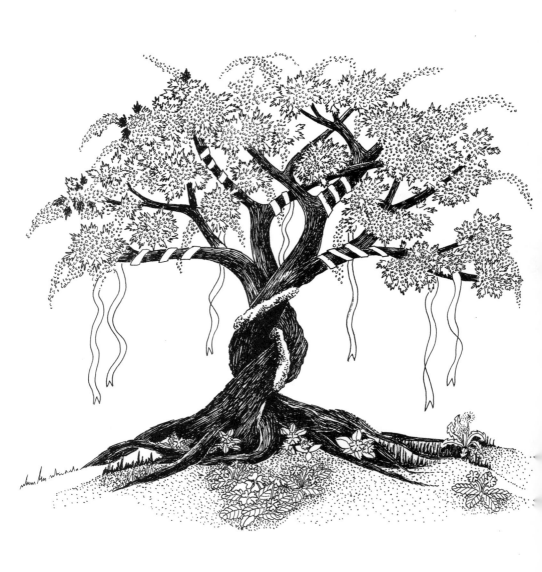

*Primrose blooming under a Hawthorn tree dressed
with ribbons in celebration of Bealtaine*

spiritual transformation. It is an ideal plant to diet with at this season of fertile growth.

# BEALTAINE
## *A Time of New Beginnings*

Bealtaine, otherwise known as Beltane or May Eve, is the major fertility festival of the year. This is the time when all of Nature is rapidly growing and moving forward with rampant potency. The life force is manifesting and bursting with creativity. It is a time to celebrate the fertility of the land and of our own creative urges; a time of growth, expansion, and playfulness, when sexual forces are at their peak. In Ireland Bealtaine marks the start of summer. According to tradition, at midnight on May Eve people rise to gather flowers and boughs to decorate their homes. They do this so the Sun will see the decorations in His honor when He arises the next morning. In our Celtic Pagan past, this was the night to celebrate the union of the Horned God and the fertile Goddess. Young couples would make love outdoors in the forests and green fields, reenacting the sacred marriage between Earth and Sky to ensure the fertility of the land. Maypoles were erected and dances performed to energize the soil. Cattle were driven through the smoke of the sacred Bealtaine fire in order to protect them from disease and to bring fertility.

In modern times we kindle a sacred fire outdoors and jump the flames in order to purify, let go, and bring forth our wildness and creativity. This is the time to honor and celebrate the wild man and woman within, to take a leap into the power of our own potential. We can explore ways to connect with our wild energy and express this through dress, dance, voice, and sexuality. Bealtaine is a time to gather with likeminded others, celebrating love, creativity, and the power of Nature. Hawthorn trees (as well as Primrose) are particularly associated with this festival and for some people the timing of Bealtaine is reckoned as the day the Hawthorn first blooms. We can honor the trees by dressing them with ribbons and flowers, giving thanks and celebrating their burgeoning growth.

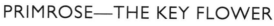

# PRIMROSE—THE KEY FLOWER
## *Primula vulgaris*

**Plant family:** Primulaceae (Primrose Family).

**Other common names:** *Samhaircin* (Irish); *Primevère* (French); *Primavera* (Spanish); *Primel* (German); *Himmelschlüssel* (German for "heaven's key"); Password; Butter Rose; Easter Rose; First Rose (*Primus,* Latin for "first," gives us *Primula* and, the first Rose of spring); Key Flower (*Primula* sp.); St Peter's Keys.

**Description:** Primrose is a hardy, deciduous perennial growing to a height of three to six inches. It has a rosette of long, crinkly leaves from which grow pale yellow flowers with deep yellow centers. These flowers arise on individual stalks in April or May, although in some sheltered places they can flower nearly all year round. Flowers are sweetly scented and have a pleasant flavor. Primrose has evolved some remarkable features for survival. The plants produce two kinds of flowers, apparently identical on the outside but inwardly quite different. One kind is known as "pin-eyed" and the other as "thrum-eyed." Even the pollen of the two flowers differs. Each individual plant has only one kind of flower, never both. This ingenious diversity of structure ensures cross-fertilization between the flowers by such long-tongued insects as bees and moths. Perhaps this unusual feature is a reflection of Primrose's role in the evolution of consciousness and the bringing together of polarities such as male and female or Earth and Sky. The plants enjoy damp conditions and individuals can live up to twenty-five years. Primroses easily form hybrids with Cowslips and Oxlips, which are closely related family members. The fruit is a capsule and the seeds are often dispersed by ants.

**Habitat:** Grassy banks, roadsides, sea cliffs, waste ground, woodlands, and fields.

**Distribution:** The genus is comprised of about 550 species with numerous hybrid groups (some have been horticultural favorites since the seventeenth century) as well as modern cultivars. Native to Europe, Asia, and Northwest Africa, European Primroses are found throughout Ireland, Britain, France, Scandinavia, and parts of Germany. In some areas they have been lost due to overharvesting. This is a protected plant in certain parts of the world, in which case the roots should not be disturbed unless it is cultivated at home. Primrose is not a North American native although it is locally established and a variety of cultivars exist throughout North America.

**Parts used:** Flowers (gathered in April–May), roots, rhizomes, and leaves (gathered in March–April). Be aware that in some countries Primrose is a protected plant and cannot be collected from the wild.

## Primrose as a Spirit Medicine

Primrose has a very clear, pure healing energy that washes away extraneous mental activity and brings feelings of deep peace. It clears obsessive thinking, instilling a calm, secure sense of connection with the Earth. At the same time it is light and playful, lifting feelings of heaviness from the heart, releasing stuck patterns, and restoring hope. When we feel stuck or confused, Primrose clears the mind and enables us to gain a new perspective. This is an essence of new beginnings. It frees creative energy, which can then flow unimpeded and without judgment. In this way Primrose can open up a huge surge of creativity, facilitating major change in people's lives and helping them in their quest for wholeness. When Primrose appears in a healing session it frequently heralds a time of transformation.

Many traditions work with the spirit of Primrose. As an herb of Bealtaine, it may be added to a sacred cup or cauldron or blended into an incense at Bealtaine celebrations. Primrose tea can be taken as a way to attune to the season. Contemporary Druids often use Primrose in particular as a ceremonial gift at the initiation of a Bard. Similarly, the flowers can be used for ceremonial decorations or to make a Primrose and Vervain tea. As an oil for anointing, Primrose flowers may be combined with Vervain. For Druids, Primrose represents creativity and rebirth while Vervain is held to stimulate inspiration. In Nordic tradition, Primrose is sacred to Freya (Goddess of Love and Beauty) and may be used in her rituals.

## Primrose as a Flower Essence

**Key words to describe this essence:**
Inner transformation; irrevocable change; initiation.

Primrose flower essence offers a key to inner transformation and rebirth. The stuck becomes unstuck and the blocked begins to move. Helpful when we feel immobilized or caught in a recurring pattern, this essence helps us to transform our attitudes and behaviors. A catalyst for major change and the clearing of obstacles, it supports us as we move into a new, expanded phase. There is no going back. Primrose is an essence of initiation.*

### *Primrose in Folklore and History*

As a spring flower, Primrose has long been considered to have special powers. An herb of Bealtaine, it is associated with the lusty currents of the season and the growing life force of fertility. In the language of flowers, Primrose is a symbol of the joys of youth. The phrase "the Primrose path" or "the path of pleasure" is associated with lust. Shakespeare made use of this phrase in *Hamlet* in 1602:

> *Doe not as some ungracious Pastors doe,*
> *Shew me the steepe and thorny way to Heaven;*
> *Whilst like a puft and reckless Libertine*
> *Himselfe the Primrose path of dalliance treads.*

In ancient Greece, Primrose was named *Paralisos* after a young man who languished away after the death of his sweetheart, Melicerta. Tree spirits (dryads) are said to pick Primroses at the new moon and in Christianity the Primrose is dedicated to several saints. In Ireland, Primroses are known as faerie flowers, and if a child eats Primroses he or she will see fairies. Also in Ireland and in other parts of Europe, yellow flowers and green branches are traditionally used as decoration and protection for the house and cattle at Bealtaine. Primrose has long been one of the favorite flowers for this. In some parts of Ireland this custom became Christianized, and Primroses are now used to decorate the May altar, dedicated to our Blessed Mary.

---

*This description refers to the specific flower essence made at Derrynagittah during the Spring Equinox 2008.

As mentioned earlier, Primrose is known as the Key Flower and has also been called *Himmelschlüssel* (Heaven's Key). It is a plant highly prized by Druids. In the past, Druidesses carried Primroses as a protection from evil and Druids used Primrose body oil as a cleanser and purifier. The ancient poem "The Chair of Taliesin" describes the initiation of a bard with a drink made from Primroses and Vervain. The plant is also mentioned by Nikolai Tolstoy in *The Coming of the King*:

> *Gwydion it was who with great magic from his wand of*
> *enchantment*
> *Flung fire among the nine forms of elements, so that they*
> *combined into*
> *A wondrous growth: essence of rich soils, water of the*
> *ninth wave,*
> *Primroses of the hillside, bloom of woods and trees.*

Primrose Hill in England is held to be one of the most sacred sites in London. It was originally called Barrow Hill being named after the tumulus on its western side.* In the past the hill was covered with Primroses every spring. In 1792 it became the location for the ceremony marking the public proclamation of the Druid Revival, reflecting the ongoing role that the Primrose plays in Druidry.

A wide variety of traditional herbal uses for Primrose have been reported over the centuries. The whole plant had a reputation for relieving nerve pain and helping rheumatism. It was thought as well to be a successful treatment for paralysis, convulsions, vertigo, and dizziness. The squeezed juice of the leaves mixed with gin was said to ward off strokes. The German healer Saint Hildegard von Bingen (1098–1179) used Primrose as a "happy-maker"† for melancholia, recommending that a compress of Primroses be bandaged on the heart overnight. Primrose may well be the plant that Roman naturalist Pliny the Elder (77 CE) referred to as the

---

*A tumulus is a mound of earth or stones raised over a grave or graves.

†Wighard Strehlow and Gottfried Hertzka, *Hildegard of Bingen's Medicine* (Rochester, Vt.: Bear & Company, 1988), 81–82.

"plant of the twelve (greater) gods"* that cures every disease if ingested in water. Some of these ancient reports may refer to other *Primula* species, such as Cowslip, which has similar properties to Primrose.

## Primrose in Contemporary Herbal Medicine

Primrose flowers make an excellent sedative and are particularly helpful for insomnia if the mind is overactive. The flowers reduce pain and spasm, relieving nervous headaches and calming restlessness and irritability. They can bring a gentle relief of the anxiety associated with nervous irritability. In all these cases, good results can be obtained by drinking an infusion of the fresh flowers, either three times daily or one cup before bed for insomnia. As few as five flowers per cup of water can be sufficient for some people. The flowers can also be made into a tincture by soaking them in alcohol for a minimum of two weeks. Use 1 part flowers to 5 parts alcohol going by either weight or volume. Tincture dosage is ½ teaspoon to 1 teaspoon (2.5–5 ml) three times daily.

The leaves have a milder sedative action but are nonetheless helpful to reduce nervous irritability if flowers are not available. My preferred use of the leaves is to make an ointment for healing wounds or ulcers. In this case they combine well with the leaves of Plantain (*Plantago lanceolata*), another exceptional wound healer. Crushed fresh Primrose leaves (or Primrose and Plantain together) can also be applied directly to a wound to speed up healing.

The root and rhizome can make a potent expectorant and demulcent, removing excess mucus while soothing and protecting inflamed, irritated internal tissue. This works primarily by virtue of the saponin content, which triggers a reflex in the digestive tract and thereby initiates the release of respiratory mucus. Root and rhizome make a powerful cough remedy, especially if the cough is nonproductive. Therefore they can help in the treatment of conditions such as bronchitis, tracheitis, and whooping cough. Primrose root and rhizome will soothe and calm excessive irritability while causing an

*Pliny the Elder, *Naturalis Historia*, book XXV, Chapter IX, and book XXVI, chapter LXVII.

effective release of mucus from the respiratory tract. Plant material should be placed in a pan of cold water (½ oz. to 20 fl. oz.) brought slowly to a boil, and simmered for ten minutes, uncovered. This decoction can be taken in wineglassful doses (up to five daily) or made into syrup by combining with sugar or honey (10 oz. sugar or honey to 20 fl. oz. of decoction). One or two teaspoons of syrup can be taken several times over the day. This can also be made into a tincture of 1 part plant material to 5 parts alcohol in doses of 1 teaspoon (5 ml) three times daily.

In contemporary herbal medicine, Primrose tends to be less commonly used than Cowslip, which some herbalists consider to have a broader range of action. From my experience, I find Primrose flowers ideal for their sedative and pain-relieving effects, particularly for sensitive individuals. The flowers make an excellent combination with Cowslip root if a strong expectorant action is needed.

## Additional Uses of Primrose

Primrose has a vast range of culinary uses. Flowers can be crystallized and petals can be used to make wine or added to flavor drinks and preserves. Flowers and leaves can be included in springtime salads, the flowers mixed with rice or other dishes, and the leaves cooked as a vegetable. At one time, Primula stew or "Primrose potage" was popular in England.

Be aware that some of the popular cultivated Primroses (*Primula obconica* and *Primula praetensis*) can cause an itchy dermatitis on contact for susceptible skin types. These cultivars are not suitable for internal use.

## PLANT DIETING WITH PRIMROSE

*After setting your sacred intention and choosing which plant to diet, in this case Primrose, it is time to harvest the plants and prepare your elixir. Below you will find recipes for two Primrose elixirs that I made for ceremonial plant diets at Derrynagittah. I have described the instructions that I received from Primrose for making these two elixirs. When making your own elixir you will need to listen carefully to the plants and let them guide you in making the perfect elixir for carrying out your intent. See chapter 4 for more complete information on harvesting plants and preparing the elixir.*

*When undertaking a plant diet, it is important to prepare yourself for several days in advance with a period of physical and spiritual purification. At Derrynagittah we make specific cleansing and dietary recommendations for each plant diet. You will find suggested preparations for the Primrose diet below.*

## 🌿 MAKING THE PRIMROSE ELIXIR

For all the elixir recipes in this book I have expressed the majority of ingredients in terms of parts of a whole. This is to avoid giving the impression of any requirement for fixed amounts and to encourage readers to make whatever amount of elixir is appropriate for themselves or their group. In most recipes you will notice that certain ingredients (notably vibrational essences) are listed with a specific quantity. In these cases, the amount is NOT proportional to the total amount of elixir and represents a quantity simply added to the whole. This is an intuitive, guided choice and the amount can remain the same, regardless of total quantity; that is, the same number of drops of essence can be added, whether to 20 oz. of elixir or 2 gallons. As already stated, these are sample recipes and you are encouraged to devise your own.

*Elixir I*
- 3 parts Primrose and Betony (*Stachys betonica*) decoction
    - I part Primrose (flowers, leaves, and roots)
    - 5 parts water
    - 7 Betony leaves
- I part Rosewater
- I teaspoon extra virgin olive oil
- 7 drops Primrose flower essence
- I part Rye alcohol

**Amount of elixir taken at diet:** Six servings of 2 tablespoons and 2 teaspoons (40 ml) for each person

This was the elixir for our first plant-diet ceremony and for its making I was given precise instructions from Spirit to pick Primroses on Good Friday morning and to start making the decoction in the afternoon at the time of the full moon. I was required to bring Primroses from the Burren (a limestone region of northwest Clare) as well as from east Clare where I live. All of the ingredients in the decoction were harvested fresh on the same day and decocted together. The Betony called to be included and felt particularly appropriate because it was mentioned in the Primrose recipe from Gerard's *Generall Historie of Plants* quoted at the end of chapter 1. A final maceration of all the ingredients had to be left over the two nights of the Easter weekend and pressed out on Easter Sunday.

The harvesting and making was a powerful and potent process and I still do not fully understand all that went on. There is an element of mystery involved in this work and my understanding continues to unfold. Gathering Primroses in the rocky landscape of the Burren, I was taken to ancient times. As I made my prayers and sang to the plants and the land, I knew that I was connecting to something very deep and that I was being called both to establish a solid connection and to carry a firm thread back to my home in east Clare. As I prepared the elixir throughout the time of the full moon, I felt Primrose dredging the unconscious realms, diving deep into the darkness and drawing up as much as she could to dance with the golden Light of cosmic energies available on Easter Sunday. I felt an overwhelming sense of freedom and that indeed Primrose was carrying the key to the gates of Tir na N'Og, the Land of Eternal Youth.

## Elixir 2

- ◈ 3 parts infusion of Primrose (flowers and leaves) and Betony (leaves)
- ◈ 3 parts decoction of Primrose root
- ◈ 1 part Rosewater
- ◈ 7 drops Kuthumi Quintessence*
- ◈ 7 drops Primrose flower essence
- ◈ 1 part Rye alcohol

---

*Kuthumi Quintessence is a liquid preparation made by Aura-Soma, U.K. Quintessences are made using herbs in an ethanol base. They are connected to Spiritual Masters and invoke positive energies from color. The Kuthumi Quintessence puts us in touch with the Master Kuthumi, who is exemplified by Saint Francis of Assisi. It carries love and wisdom and nurtures the angelic-human-devic connection, helping us attune to plants and connect with devas, angels, faeries, and other beings.

**Amount of elixir taken at diet:** Nine servings of 2 tablespoons (30 ml) for each person

During this harvesting a cuckoo bird led me around our land, singing a signal of two notes each time I was to pick some Primroses. Fewer flowers were needed than usual but the locations were important. I became very aware of the sounds of the birds and the insects, the wind in the trees, and the flowing of the river. I was told not to sing but I was given a tune to play on my xylophone. I was conscious of how the Primroses were behaving like receptor dishes, picking up signals from afar. I was told to leave the picked Primroses in water for a while in the third ring of the labyrinth. Here they sat in the Eastern Gateway of Initiation, connecting with Oak, Holly, Blackthorn, and up to the stars. I also picked some Vervain from the herb garden to make a version of the Bardic Cup,* which I prepared from Vervain tops and Primrose flowers, boiled in water and flavored with fruit juice.

##  PREPARATION FOR THE PRIMROSE PLANT DIET

### General Preparations
For three days prior to the diet take NO refined sugar, added salt, meat or dairy products, strong spices, coffee, alcohol, or fermented foods. Avoid oils apart from olive oil. Do not engage in sexual activity.

### Gentle Liver Cleanse
In addition to the general preparations, for the Primrose diets we recommend a gentle liver cleanse for three days prior to the ceremony. Take 1 to 3 tablespoons of extra virgin olive oil with three times that amount of fresh lemon juice on rising each morning. Follow this with two glasses of the juice of a half lemon and hot water. Then either fast or wait one hour before having a simple breakfast of something like oats, seeds, nuts, and/or fruit.

### Food during the Primrose Diet
For those not fasting we recommend oats and almonds.

---

*The Bardic Cup represents a Celtic initiatory cauldron, as alluded to in the ancient poem "The Chair of Taliesin" (*Book of Taliesin,* vol. 13, medieval Welsh Manuscript). In our case it was offered to initiates as part of a labyrinth ceremony during the plant diet.

*Suggested Drinks*

We recommend Dandelion root decoction, Nettle tea, and either hot or cold water.

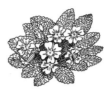

## DREAMING WITH PRIMROSE

*Through the alchemy of sacred ceremony, participants in a plant diet enter into an altered state in which they form close relationships with the plant that they are dieting. By surrendering to all that the plant offers, participants enter the dream of the plant and receive gifts that may be physical, emotional, mental, and spiritual. Many participants gain a completely new perspective on life. The relationship with the plant is deeply transformative, facilitating access to higher consciousness, guidance, and healing. In this section people who have dieted with Primrose tell the stories of their personal transformations.*

A plant initiation starts as soon as you have set your intent to participate. Sometimes this brings noticeable effects before ingesting the elixir. One participant, Linda, became aware of the physical effects two days in advance of the ceremony:*

> *The days before coming, I felt ill and had to stay in bed Thursday and Friday. I had bad pains in my bones and muscles and I had no energy. I kept getting really hot, which is not like me. I knew it was the Primrose.*

After first taking the elixir, Linda rapidly moved into an altered state and during the weekend she experienced strong connections with both the Earth and the stars. She felt she received much healing and was aware that this was collective as well as personal:

---

*Some names have been changed to protect the privacy of participants.

*When I first took the elixir I felt the Primrose very strong, so strong I felt I might throw up. I cannot remember all that happened while doing the light wheels. At one point I felt I was the Earth and I felt Primroses growing around me. I felt my body was dropping and jumping and I felt healing taking place. I was crying and I do not know why, it just came. There was a connection with the constellation Cassiopeia. Then my right contact lens moved in my eye and I went out on our trip to meet the Primrose with one eye blurry and one fine. At the blessing of the Primrose I knew if I did not get up when I was finished I would have been taken somewhere else by the Primrose. I had to pull myself back. I went to the area below the herb garden and although I do not remember much of what happened, there were little tiny beings and the roots of the tree were moving, full of life. I lay on the ground and drifted off somewhere. I visited Sirius the oak tree on the way back. I was in a dreamlike state and I had no concept of time. Part of the time I felt I was under the earth, in the earth, and sometimes I was the Primrose. There was a beautiful Light coming from it. There was a connection with the stars, both the Primrose's connection and my connection. That felt really emotional. I was conscious of doing this for the collective as well as for myself. At the very end I saw a pure white candle with a strong flame and loads of hands raised up with white Light coming from them. The last time I took the elixir I felt very joyous and could feel it going down my arms and into my body. It felt good.*

For many participants, there was an immediate effect from first drinking the Primrose elixir. As one woman commented, "From the first drinking it felt very potent. I had a headache and felt a desire to lie down and just really be with the Primrose." Another described "a lot of spasms in my body when first taking the Primrose."

Mary Teresa's experience took her back in time:

*As soon as I took the Primrose elixir I felt I was pulled back somewhere. I was back to when I was a tiny child living with my Grandmother and I felt I relived all those years and all the happy memories. I experienced so much joy and happiness and could see and feel her like she was. I really loved her.*

*Then I was yanked away, living with my mother and father and sisters. I did not want to be there. I kept day dreaming of being with my grandmother and wanted to go back to her. I felt I was living with strangers. The whole day I was coming in and out of this, being happy with her, and then being without her and dreaming of being with her again.*

Later, Mary Teresa found that Primrose was helping her to stay in her body:

*My obstacle was that I was constantly escaping out of my body when challenges came. One of my ancestors was there and kept pressing my energy body back into my body. The Primrose was in me and all around, sealing it in place. I was stamping my feet and could feel the two coming together.*

## The Radiance of Primrose

Typical images were of the "beautiful light" and "stunning radiance" emitted by Primrose. Laura had this to say:

*This is a very powerful radiant being. I'm almost afraid of its radiance and it shows me the possible and potential radiance that I carry and can shine forth. What a huge responsibility to be true to your radiance. The theme is not to get distracted from your soul's path.*

## Healing and Letting Go

Many people reported receiving healing. Patrick said:

*I had a very physical experience. I kept waking up coughing and really having trouble swallowing because it felt like knives in my throat. It was like I was making lots of saliva but actually it was the Primrose and it was soothing all of my throat. A big healing took place in my throat and chest. Today my chest feels much better.*

Joan met the spirit of Primrose on a mountaintop:

*She was beautiful, as was the place. It was the colors of Primrose. She spoke to me and asked me to lie down on a bed of Primroses and she gave me a healing.*

Later, while breathing with Primrose during the GreenBreath, Joan transformed a major fear that came from her great grandfather:

*When I met my fear it was about being ridiculed and kept separate. I realized this is stuff from my great grandfather and it had come up for me a lot lately. When I was giving this stuff back to my great grandfather I felt really guilty. I found it very difficult to do, but I did it. I thanked him and I felt him move on after that. The whole energy shifted. Now I feel part of life and I feel excited about engaging in it. I also realize that the little Primrose helped bring me to that process.*

For Dalton, the GreenBreath involved an intense letting go:

*It was probably the most intense experience I have ever had, more intense than any healing I have had before. I felt really unclean during it. I was in floods of sweat and wanted to take off my clothes. It felt like I was getting a healing and it felt like something disgusting was getting released. When we started breathing with the Primrose I felt like I did not need to get its approval. We felt equal and that felt really good. I kept bursting into tears because of how pure it was. I feel now my love for nature and its love for me is locked inside forever. Tears of joy came and I kept getting an image of a tree, the kind of thing you would draw as a child. I could see the image of the labyrinth in it. I felt amazing afterward. I felt great healing.*

In one of my own dreams, I experienced a part of myself being returned:

*In one of the dreams I had during the night I was lying next to a young woman with short, cropped hair. She was unconscious, lying in a hospital bed, looking pale and thin, and wearing a pale hospital gown. She looked like someone who had been either on chemotherapy or in a concentration camp. Then Mary Teresa and I were on either side of the bed singing to her. After a while we were joined by a host of spirit beings all singing to this young woman who remained unconscious and they said to me, "Don't worry, she will return." I felt she was some aspect of myself. I feel very grateful that the Primrose (and Mary Teresa) have helped in the process of bringing her back.*

## Primrose as the Key Flower

Images of keys and doorways commonly arose when dieting with Primrose. As Laura commented:

*Primrose seems to hold the key to unlock the door to inner riches and treasures, one's true essential nature. She asks for us to wake up—wake up and open to these gifts.*

The following is Laura's account from a rattle journey with Primrose:

*Lela took me to a tiny little cottage. I asked her how I was to get in. She said you have to make yourself small. I asked how to do that and she said to listen to the rattle. I became small like an insect to get into this very tiny cottage. There was an old woman inside and I asked if she was the spirit of Primrose. "Lord no," she said, "I'm to give you a cup of Primrose tea." She got out these tiny cups and gave me tea. When I finished she took a big key off the wall and told me to follow her. I followed her out to her garden where there was a big wooden door rounded at the top. At some point the sound had changed and I asked her about this. She said I was now in the land of the faeries and that many things are different here. She said, "You do know Primrose is of the faeries." Then she unlocked the door. When the door opened a dazzling Light came out. When I went inside there were staffs and wands with crystals in them all over the place, lots of gold too. This beautiful faery queen appeared and asked if I would like one of the wands. She picked a beautiful wand/staff with a clear quartz crystal point*

*on the end and embedded jewels and stones on the shaft. There was gold*
*spiralling around it. It was so beautiful. I asked if I needed a wand/staff in*
*physical form and she said it may come to me someday. As I thanked her*
*and was about to leave she said, "Now you must serve me well." I agreed*
*and went out the door, back to the cottage, and then back with Lela. What*
*a beautiful journey!*

## The Land of Faery

Entering the land of faery is another common thread, echoed by Mary's
account:

> *When sitting with the Primrose she took me inside the flower like going*
> *down a shoot at a swimming pool and I landed in a beautiful blue sea with*
> *the sun shining down. I had entered the faery world. It felt like leaving*
> *something behind and heading for a new beginning. There has been such a*
> *lot of faery energy present for me all weekend. It's very childlike. I feel like*
> *a child being reborn. I really enjoyed doing some paintings.*

Maeve had a similar experience and found this led to a great feeling
of safety:

> *When we went out on the land to be with the Primrose I felt such connection*
> *with so many plants, such a feeling of Oneness and connection with the*
> *faeries. I became very tiny and found I was walking lightly on the land, like*
> *a tiny child, a faery child, completely filled with awe and wonder at the*
> *immense beauty around me. I traveled down the center of the Primrose*
> *flower, through her delicate watery stem, up through the lush green of her*
> *leaf, savoring and resonating with the vibration of the green. Then I went*
> *down into her roots and drank from the Earth, being nourished by this*
> *mineral-rich fluid. Later on I traveled again through her calyx, entering*
> *that fertile place. In my tiny form I was enfolded by her green leaf. It closed*
> *around me like a cocoon. I was a chrysalis waiting to emerge. It was green*
> *and warm in there. I was held in total safety.*

## Dismemberment

Dismemberment describes the process of breaking down the old in order to be reformed in a new way. It is a centuries-old method of initiation used in numerous cultures all over the planet, a method whereby the ego dies so that one can become more one's true self. During a spiritual dismemberment, a person will experience a vision where he or she is literally dismembered by Spirit. For instance, this could entail being eaten by an animal, cut open, consumed by fire, or stripped to the bone by the pecking of birds. Spirit will regularly place crystals or healing plants inside the body before it is reformed. Sometimes surgery is carried out by Spirit taking on plant, human, or animal form.

Dismemberment is a common experience when working deeply with plant spirits, especially during a plant initiation ceremony. A dismemberment oftentimes occurs as a spontaneous vision, for example in a dream or during a healing or meditation. Sometimes as part of a plant initiation I facilitate an intentional dismemberment journey. This can be particularly appropriate with Primrose. Initiates are encouraged to trust the plant, to surrender to the process, and to know that they will indeed be reformed in a way of beauty. In the following, the intention was to meet with the Primrose spirit and ask for a dismemberment. Below, Laura describes how the dismemberment made her ready to fully receive the power in the wand given earlier:

> During the dismemberment journey when the little old lady unlocked the door, it was dark inside except for one candle. I couldn't see Primrose. She told me to get on the table. I said I was afraid. She didn't know why because I would get put back together even better than I was before. She said she would cut out the lazy part that leads to not being authentic, the part that needs to take time out to be with plants and Spirit instead of it being a part of my natural flow. Tulsi, Artemisia, and Hawthorn came to be with me during the dismemberment surgery. It didn't really hurt. They took all my parts in a basket to the stream at my home to make sure I was put back together properly. Tulsi, my soul, Hawthorn, my heart, and Artemisia, my energy body made sure I was put back together. When I was back together again I was in the land of the faery queen. She was her

*beautiful self again. She gave me an identical wand as before. She said this one had the power in it. When she said this, the pad I was lying on literally bounced up and down. She said she knew I wasn't ready for the power-filled wand before but now I was ready.*

Joan's dismemberment gave her access to awesome powers:

*I first went to a stream in the woods where I live. From there I was taken to meet the Primrose at a mountain stream. I lay down and three wolves arrived. One took my head and the others an arm each. There was no blood and I did not feel afraid. Each ran away with a limb. It was to feed their cubs. I felt through these limbs the love and tenderness they had for their cubs. A grizzly bear came and took the rest of my body. I could feel its strength and physical power. A black panther took my right leg and dragged it up a tree. An eagle took my left leg and carried it to its chicks and fed them with it. With each animal I had now become part of them. I felt in awe of them and the powers that I was a part of. It was a beautiful experience.*

## *Primrose as a Bridge*

In this final account from Laura, which describes the power of love and the importance of dreaming, Primrose explains how she can be a bridge between lands. Primrose as a bridge is another recurring theme, a personal reminder for me of how Primrose links Derrynagittah to Sweetwater,* Islay, and so many other locations. It also reflects my experiences from making Primrose elixirs:

*In the final journey I followed a yellow brick road with Tulsi, Artemisia, and Hawthorn to the Emerald City castle. Faery queen Primrose greeted us. Everything had twinkles of light on it. She took me to a solarium that again was light filled with crystalline twinkling lights. She told me she could make a bridge to any land just the way she has made a bridge between*

---

*Sweetwater Sanctuary is Pam Montgomery's center for healing and education in southern Vermont.

*Sweetwater and Derrynagittah. I asked, "Even if you don't grow in the
particular land I want to go to?" She said this is dreamtime space. She is
the spirit of Primrose and her gifts are outside of time and space. She also
told me that I need to give equal accord to the dreamtime space as I do to
ordinary reality as so much can happen in the dreamtime. Something can't
manifest until you dream it. She reminded me that my power is my love.*

## Expanding Consciousness and the Message of Love

In the next account, Primrose is seen to be bringing a message of love and
Oneness to the planet. This initiate receives a new awareness of what love
is and how she can embody that. She is also given some techniques for
learning detachment:

*I wake up feeling huge mental struggles going on. I can feel myself detaching
from the mind and its games—the "mind maze." I see my mind and its
jumbled thoughts and obsessions in a box and I am pulling back from the
box, detaching, pulling back to a place of peace and joy and excitement.
Traveling with the music I find myself going to places of ecstasy with the
sound. My mind keeps fighting to come back and I make the box bigger.
All the mind maze stuff continues inside the box. There is also a box for
my emotions. I am pulling away and observing these responses and it gives
me a great sense of freedom. This is a place of pure Spirit or consciousness
and I'm wondering why I don't stay here all the time? Why don't I make
a new choice? Choose not to stay in the mind maze? I am taken back to
when I was eleven or twelve, when following a spiritual experience I tried
to love all the others in the world unconditionally, but had no clue how to
boundary myself. Then feeling abused and taken advantage of, I decided
that love wasn't possible in this way, that I couldn't survive in the world like
this. Now I can see that I had the wrong idea about what unconditional
love is. I can see that love is possible and love is safe. This makes my heart
feel liberated. Relief floods through me and I feel my heart so expanded.
The Primrose fills my heart and steadies it. She is in every light wheel but
especially strong in my heart. She is dancing with my seventh wheel, yellow
and violet together. I see her dancing with the Ayahausca vine, Primrose*

*flowers encircling the vine. They are working together. The message of the Ayahausca is also being spread by the Primrose. They are sister plants, both from the stars. It's a message that teaches about love and Oneness, love with detachment. The Primrose flowers also go inside and help to calm the mind. They tell me to keep closing the door to the mind maze. It's a physical door. I see myself repeatedly leaving that box, getting tempted back, then leaving again. I will keep practicing.*

Her final comments provide a useful summing up:

*This has been a profound initiation for me. I feel we have unlocked a major gateway, that the Primrose opens our vision and shows us the illusions we create. She cuts ties to the past and raises our consciousness so that we can see into the hollow hills and connect with the faeries and reach out to the stars and remember who we are. Now I am more relaxed and present, like I have expanded into myself and it is very freeing.*

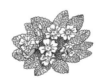

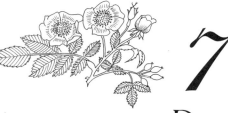

# 7

# Dog Rose 🌹
# Summer Solstice
## *Opening the Heart*

*D*og Rose is a delight of early summer, dotting the June hedgerows with her clear, bright blooms (see color plate 5). Ruled by both Venus and the moon, she has a feminine nature and her five-petaled flowers mark her as a plant of the Goddess.* She is associated with the element of water and with emerald and turquoise gemstones. Her delicate, heart-shaped petals range in color from pure white through palest pink to deep pink. They are easily dislodged, fluttering in the breeze like confetti at a wedding, bringing to mind a celebration of love and union. Later in the year she brightens the winter hedgerows with a mass of fertile, crimson rosehips. Paradoxically, she is at once soft and vulnerable yet fiercely strong and protective. Her delicate blossoms belie the strength and vigor of her creeping, spreading stems. Curved and reddened thorns arise on her flexible limbs, finding support and offering protection. She may appear shy but she is stronger than she might look!

Blooming at the peak of the sun's power in June, Dog Rose is associated

---

*In the lore of the Old Ways, a flower with five petals is representative of a five-pointed star and held as sacred to the Goddess.

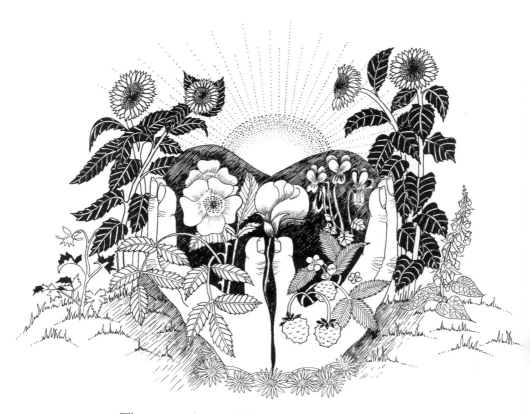

*The sun reaches its full power at the Summer Solstice.*

with the fulfillment and expansiveness of the height of summer. Her beautiful flowers express the attainment of pure, unconditional love and the ultimate flowering of Spirit. She is a perfect plant to diet with at the Summer Solstice.*

# SUMMER SOLSTICE
## Fulfillment and Manifestation

In the Northern Hemisphere, the Summer Solstice is the longest day and the shortest night of the year. In the west of Ireland there are only a few hours of darkness. The energy of Grandfather Sun is peaking at the height of its power. In the past, people stayed up all night on Midsummer's Eve to watch the sunrise and celebrate the longest day. Bonfires were lit on hills at midnight and people danced around the fires and leapt the flames to rid themselves of bad luck and to assure abundance and the fertility of the land. Livestock were blessed with blazing herbs from the fire and flaming torches were taken sunwise around field and home. Sacred trees were dressed with flowers and ribbons and it was a time of games and feasting. Sun Gods and Goddesses were honored, such as the goddess Áine in County Limerick where today people still pay homage at her sacred hill.

The Summer Solstice is a time to celebrate what has manifested. We celebrate the abundant growth that has occurred in Nature as well as the attainment and fulfillment that has occurred in our lives. It is time to enjoy what we have and who we are. We fully express our uniqueness and we call on the strength and power of the sun to charge our intentions. At the same time, the Wheel of the Year is turning and from now on the days will shorten. A transformation is taking place. We prepare to return to the darkness of the inner worlds, activated and strengthened by the peaking energy.

---

*All Roses have a good deal in common so some of the information in this chapter inevitably applies to all types of rose. For example, all Roses connect to the heart. However, within the general Rose community, each species has its own unique personality and spirit. Any Roses could be appropriately dieted at midsummer, it depends what calls to you. Here in Ireland, Dog Rose is the strongest wild-rose energy we have, and this which makes it the obvious choice for our plant diets.

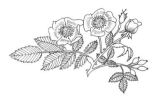

# DOG ROSE—EMBLEM OF LOVE
*Rosa canina*

**Plant family:** Rosaceae (Rose Family).

**Other common names:** Wild Rose; Briar; Hip-tree.

**Description:** A rambling, deciduous shrub with arching stems, curved thorns, and divided leaves up to two inches long. Flowers are fragrant pink or white. Bright scarlet ovoid hips are borne in autumn.

**Habitat:** Hedgerows; woodland; scrub.

**Distribution:** Widespread throughout Europe, this is the most common wild Rose in Ireland and Britain. Introduced to North America from Europe, this species is found on the east coast from Quebec to North Carolina and west to Kansas. On the west coast it is found from British Columbia to California and east to Utah.

**Related Species:** About one hundred species of Rose exist in northern temperate regions.

**Parts used:** Flowers (gathered in early to midsummer), hips (harvested in autumn), and less often, leaves (harvested in spring or early summer).

## Dog Rose as a Spirit Medicine

Dog Rose carries an exquisitely beautiful energy of unconditional love. As a practitioner it can be quite ecstatic to feel this energy pouring through and to experience the love that is present. I am continually awestruck by the gentle strength that Dog Rose offers. She has so much power and yet she is completely gentle and yielding, never pushing further than a person is ready to go. With constancy, dedication, and loving acceptance, Dog Rose melts away our pain and stuck beliefs, layer by layer, never giving up on us, willing to go the distance however long it takes.

Dog Rose goes deep into the heart, as deeply as we will allow. Typically, we experience an enormous sense of relief in the heart when we let in Dog Rose. She restores the joyful inner child and helps with trust issues. Dog Rose soothes and softens the heart, transforming feelings of loss, betrayal, grief, heartbreak, guilt, and shame—anything that keeps us from accepting and loving ourselves. She teaches how to manifest love in the world and how to learn the balance of giving and receiving. She gives with joy and without expecting anything in return and fully receives the abundance offered by the Universe.

At the same time, Dog Rose can bring robust protection, especially for the heart. She brings teachings about boundaries and in healing sessions I have seen how she sometimes weaves a protective shield around the heart or the auric field. Dog Rose carries all aspects of the Goddess, the ability to love, nurture, and see the beauty in all things. She can assist those who seek to connect with the Goddess in any of her forms. Symbolizing love and the sacred marriage of God and Goddess, Dog Rose is a particularly appropriate plant to call upon at weddings and at Bealtaine as well as at the Summer Solstice.

## Dog Rose as a Flower Essence

**Key words to describe this essence:**
Oneness; unity consciousness.

This essence carries the vibration of Oneness. It heals feelings of separation and helps us to become conscious of our connection with all other beings: minerals, plants, animals, humans, ourselves, planet Earth and beyond, and ultimately of our connection with Source. It makes ending the separation a priority and reminds us that we are all One, making it helpful if we feel alone or separated from Source. In addition, Dog Rose essence supports the feminine and opens the heart.

## Dog Rose in Folklore and History

Dog Rose, like all species of Rose, has inspired people for centuries as an emblem of love and beauty. No other flower has quite the same effect. Roses are sacred to Aphrodite and Venus, goddesses of Love, and are seen to represent the vulva. They are regarded as aphrodisiacs and it is said that Cleopatra seduced Anthony while standing knee deep in Roses. The Romans used Rose petals to decorate their banqueting halls and to fill the place with their enchanting scent. Sometimes guests were showered with Rose petals and it is held that at one banquet so many petals showered down from the ceiling that some of the guests were suffocated. At Roman gatherings when a Rose hung on the ceiling it meant that nothing said at the meeting could be repeated outside. Still today the plaster ornament in the center of the ceiling is known as the ceiling Rose. Roman brides and bridegrooms were crowned with Roses, as were images of Venus, Cupid, and Bacchus. Some of the many other deities associated with the Rose include Blodeuwedd, Christ, Demeter, Eros, Freya, Hathor, Hymen, and Isis.* In Ireland Rose petals were scattered at weddings to ensure a happy marriage.

Rose symbolizes mystical or divine love and is emblematic of the heart or mystical center of being. Rose buds have been used as prayer beads and the modern day rosary was originally a string of rose buds. Avicenna, the Persian philosopher and scientist, is thought to have been the first to make Rose water in the tenth century. The Rose has long been valued for its healing abilities as well as its beauty and fragrance. Rosehips have been found at prehistoric dwelling sites in Britain, suggesting a very long history of human use. Herbalists of old recognized the Rose as an important plant. Sixteenth century herbalist John Gerard said:

> The distilled water of roses is good for strengthening the heart and refreshing the spirits and likewise for all things that require a gentle cooling . . . it mitigateth the pain of the eies proceeding a hot cause, bringeth sleep, which also the fresh roses themselves provoke through their sweet and pleasant smell.†

And Culpepper said of Rose medicines, "To write at large of every one of these would swell my book too big."‡

In European folk tradition Rose has been extensively used in love spells. One method to attract a lover was to remove all your clothes and jewelry

---

*See appendix 1 on pages 276–78 for deity descriptions.
†John Gerard, *Gerard's Herbal: The History of Plants*, reprint ed., edited by Marcus Woodward (London: Senate, 1994), 273.
‡Nicholas Culpeper, *Culpeper's Complete Herbal and English Physician*, reprint ed. (London: Harvey Sales, 1981).

and walk through a garden scattering Rose petals as you walk. It is said that your lover will soon appear. Other methods that are perhaps more practical in a cold climate include adding Rose buds to your bath water or placing petals in a red cloth bag and pinning it under your clothes.

## Dog Rose in Contemporary Herbal Medicine

This is the flower of love and has a wonderful affinity with the human heart. As an herbal medicine I primarily use Rose petals in tea, tinctures, or syrup to heal, calm, and support the heart in cases of emotional pain, grief, anxiety, and depression. Rose has a gentle softening and restorative action on the heart, being especially helpful if a person feels heartbreak or a lack of love. Both petals and hips (the latter to a lesser extent) are uplifting and calming for the nervous system, relieving insomnia and calming heart palpitations. Rose petals combine well with Hawthorn (also from the Rose family) if the heart needs extra physical strengthening.

Rose petals and hips offer support for the immune system and can help fight infection in the digestive tract and reduce excess stomach acid (hips being preferential for these uses). They are cooling and astringent and when taken as a tea they reduce heat in the body, clear toxins, and bring down fevers. They are also mildly diuretic, thereby assisting in the elimination of wastes through the urinary system. An infusion can be used to relieve cold and flu symptoms, sore throat, runny nose, and blocked bronchial tubes. The astringent effect can be helpful for diarrhea, colitis, and gastritis.

Rose petals also have an affinity for the female reproductive system. The astringent and decongestant effects can be useful for heavy or irregular periods, infertility, painful periods, and uterine fibroids. Rose enhances sexual desire in both men and women and has a balancing action, which makes it helpful for premenstrual syndrome and menopausal anxiety.

Rosehips contain large amounts of vitamin C as well as vitamins A, B, and K. This makes them useful for vitamin deficiency, convalescence, debility, and those prone to infection. Both Rose hips and petals are particularly suited to children.

An infusion of the petals can be used to bathe sore and inflamed eyes, as a rinse for mouth ulcers and inflamed gums, and as a douche for vaginal discharge. The infusion also makes a useful wash for radiation burns and can be used as a lotion or made into a cream to apply after radiation damage. For instance, this can be beneficial to heal burns after a radiation treatment for cancer, which is also a time when it can be especially helpful to receive the loving support of the Rose.

In addition, the petals, whether as a tea or distilled as Rosewater, make a fragrant, antiseptic skin toner and cleanser for blemishes, spots, and rashes. Rosewater is particularly useful for dry, mature, inflamed, and sensitive skins. Rose has an affinity for pregnancy when a Rose petal bath or a gentle Rose oil massage can be highly beneficial to mother and unborn child.

### Additional Uses of Dog Rose

Many spiritual traditions use Rose petals for blessing. I like to use them to give heart blessings to plants and trees, finding that their heart-shaped petals create an instant connection with my own heart. Rosehips are traditionally used in making wine, vinegars, and preserves. They are also made into syrup as a nutritional supplement, especially for babies, and the powdered hips are made into pills. Extracts from Rosehips are added to vitamin C tablets.

Petals are distilled for oil. Both Rosewater and essential oil are extensively used as perfume. The essential oil is helpful for all emotional problems of the heart and the beautiful fragrance of Rose offers its own potent medicine. Diluted Rose oil makes a wonderful anointing oil for the energetic heart center, being applied over the heart area to connect with the emotions and bring healing. Rosewater gives flavor to confectionery (notably turkish delight), desserts, sorbets, mousses, and jellies. Petals are crystallized and made into syrups and preserves.

Rose petal tincture is traditionally used to mend a broken heart. For this you should pick rose petals at noon on a sunny day, talking to the plant all the time, explaining your intentions and asking to be shown which flowers to gather. Call down blessings from the Goddess as you work and after picking, give thanks and offer a gift as a blessing. Fill a glass jar with the petals, cover with vodka, close the jar, and leave it in a dark place for two to four weeks, shaking occasionally, and acknowledging the beauty within. Strain through muslin or a fine sieve. Take 20 drops once or twice daily, calling to the spirit of Rose to bless you and mend your heart.

# PLANT DIETING WITH DOG ROSE

*After choosing to diet Dog Rose, it is time to harvest the plants and prepare your elixir. Below you will find recipes for two Dog Rose elixirs that I made at Derrynagittah. I have described the instructions that I received from Dog Rose for making these two elixirs. When making your own elixir you will need to listen carefully to the plants and let them guide you. See chapter 4 for more complete information on harvesting plants and preparing the elixir.*

*In advance of your plant diet it is important to prepare yourself for several days with a period of physical and spiritual purification. At Derrynagittah we make specific cleansing and dietary recommendations for each diet. You will find the recommended preparations for the Dog Rose diet below.*

## 🌿 MAKING THE DOG ROSE ELIXIR

You will notice that while most components in the elixir recipes below are expressed as parts of the whole, certain ingredients (notably vibrational essences) are listed with a specific quantity. In these cases, the amount is NOT proportional to the total amount of elixir and represents a quantity simply added to the whole. This is an intuitive, guided choice and the amount can remain the same, regardless of total quantity; that is, the same number of drops of essence can be added, whether to 20 oz. of elixir or 2 gallons.

*Elixir I*
- 2 parts decoction of Rose petals preserved in Brandy
- I part Rosehip and honey syrup

**Amount of elixir taken at diet:** Six servings of I tablespoon and 2 teaspoons (25 ml) for each person

**Important note:** The short hairs on Rosehip seeds can irritate the gastrointestinal tract. When making syrup, strain the hips to remove the irritant hairs.

For this elixir, the Rose petals were picked in May at an ancient Druidic site in the south of France and the Rosehips were picked at Derrynagittah in October.

This elixir forged a connection between France and Ireland. The petals were harvested while I was in France to teach a workshop. I had not intended to start making an elixir during this trip, but one morning I went for an early walk near to some ancient Yew trees and I came upon a most beautiful stand of Dog Roses in full bloom. Several Dog Roses had grown together in a massive clump in the center of a field. It looked like an enormous Dog Rose tree and I had never seen anything like it! The flowers fervently urged me to pick them explaining that they needed to come back to Ireland and make a connection between the lands. So it was that on the last day of the workshop I returned to the field and brought back bowlfuls of soft, fragrant petals. That evening in Avignon I made a decoction and used local brandy to preserve it. Interestingly, that trip marked the start of a strong association between Derrynagittah and France and we now host regular workshops here for French speakers. For many years I have known the Dog Rose as the overlighting deva of Derrynagittah so I am not surprised by her behavior and I am grateful for her clear guidance.

The Rosehips were picked here later that year. This time I had gone around the land specifically looking for Rosehips, going to areas where I had recently seen an abundance of scarlet hips. To my surprise there were very few remaining. I was called to a spot on the riverbank where a stunning Flame tree grows. At first I tried to ignore the call, intent on keeping focused on my quest, going to the places I believed I should. However, the call was so strong I decided to go back and honor the Flame tree with its mass of beautiful flame-colored leaves. Imagine my surprise when I realized that growing amid the Flame tree was a mature Dog Rose, resplendent with dazzling hips! How had I not seen it before? Anyway, the Dog Rose was very pleased to see me now and keen to share her fruit. Many of the hips were hanging over the riverbank, with some even touching the water. As I leaned to pick them, the smaller branches attached themselves to my jacket and pulled me close as if they were hugging me. The whole experience was intensely moving. It gave me a new understanding of Dog Rose's watery nature and I was blessed to receive a Dog Rose song, which I have subsequently sung at plant diets. The area by the Flame tree has since become one of my favorite riverside meditation spots.

### Elixir 2

- ❧ I part tincture of Rosehips in vodka
- ❧ I part cold infusion of Rose petals
- ❧ I tablespoon and I teaspoon each of two Dog Rose elixirs from previous diets
- ❧ 5 drops of Dog Rose flower essence

**Amount of elixir taken at diet:** Five servings of 2 tablespoons and 2 teaspoons (40 ml) for each person

For this elixir the Rosehips were picked during the Cosmic Convergence of September 2011, held to be a significant event in the Mayan Calendar. At that time I was reminded of the wildness of Dog Rose. I saw how the plant needs to be wild in order to be truly healthy and how I personally need to honor my own wild nature in order to be truly myself.

During the harvesting of the flowers I was struck by the transience and delicacy of the blooms; such beauty and nonattachment! They are totally present in their beauty and release it joyfully without holding on. The petals are so easily dislodged that a small gust of wind can easily take them. On that day heart-shaped petals lay all around me on the ground and were continuing to fall like a blizzard of confetti. I felt the celebration of the sacred marriage between the Lord and Lady of the land and the familiar sensation of Dog Rose softening my heart.

## 🌿 PREPARATION FOR THE DOG ROSE PLANT DIET

### General Preparations

For three days prior to the diet take NO refined sugar, added salt, meat or dairy products, strong spices, coffee, alcohol, or fermented foods. Avoid oils apart from olive oil. Do not engage in sexual activity.

### Food during the Dog Rose Diet

For those not fasting we recommend almonds, raisins, and honey.

*Suggested Drinks*

We recommend Chamomile or Lavender tea and hot or cold water.

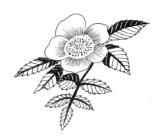

# DREAMING WITH DOG ROSE

*Through the alchemy of sacred ceremony and by surrendering to the plant, participants in a plant diet enter into an altered state in which they form close relationships with the plant that they are dieting and receive gifts that may be physical, emotional, mental, and spiritual. Many participants gain a completely new perspective on life. The relationship with the plant is deeply transformative, facilitating access to higher consciousness, guidance, and healing. In this section people who have dieted with Dog Rose tell the stories of their personal transformations.*

## *Healing and the Heart*

Healing is a recurring and major theme at every plant initiation, manifesting on all levels. When Mary attended a Dog Rose ceremony she explained that she had been suffering with back pain for several months. After drinking the elixir she reported the following:

> I lay down and experienced a sharp pain in my lower back. The only way I could handle it was by lying in the fetal position. I could feel the Dog Rose pulsating up my spine. It cleared some deep pain that day and since then my back has felt better than for months prior.

Pat also experienced physical healing from Dog Rose:

> I feel I have had a huge amount of healing this weekend. The swelling on my knee has gone right down and both my knees feel much freer. I have

*had this swelling and pain for about five years and it has been really strong for the past six months. In the GreenBreath I felt the Dog Rose freeing up parts of my body. I had a flash of acute pain in my knees at one point. My sense was that my knees were broken and that at some time in the past they had been broken as a punishment for being myself and for dancing. As I breathed I felt more and more free and that my knees weren't broken. Instead I felt a freedom going through my legs and a freedom in moving. In the last while there has been a fear about doing things in case I make my knees worse and my understanding was to let that go.*

Many participants described receiving healing for their hearts. Pat revealed:

*After I had the first drink of Dog Rose elixir I had the sense of someone cleaning out my heart with a brush. The last bit of sadness about Jenny in my heart is gone. Jenny was my second daughter and she died when she was four, when I was pregnant with Elizabeth. I realized during the GreenBreath that I have finally let go of her.*

Mary Teresa also experienced healing in her heart:

*In the GreenBreath I found myself lying in the grass with the Dog Rose all around. It merged with me. I was the plant and the plant was me. I had vines and leaves and flowers growing out of my body. It filled my insides and I could feel it moving around within. I could feel it moving in my head, behind my eyes, and in my ears. I felt it moving down my throat and my arms and legs and then it came to my heart and my heart felt heavy. I could feel a sense of grief and loss. I could feel the Rose circling my heart and as it did I felt my chest was expanding and moving. I felt myself dissolve and I no longer had a body. When I came back into my body I felt stronger and there was an old African lady there and she rubbed oils all over my body and anointed my third eye in the eight directions. She made a poultice from the flowers of the Dog Rose and she put them on my heart. She told me she could teach me much and asked, "What about your medicine name? What about beauty, love, and passion?" We sat by the fire together and she gave me something to drink, which tasted sweet of honey. Then the African man was there and she was gone. It is like they are different aspects of the same person. She is very old, patient, and kind and he is very young and demanding. He seemed very agitated with me and he started massaging parts of my body and pulling things out of my third eye and my left side. There was a steel brace around my neck and it felt very restricting. He opened it and I felt a release but there was still a fabric wrapped tightly round my neck and he cut this off. Even though this was gone I could still feel my neck restricted. He dragged me to a pool of water and told me it was the pool of reflection and asked me if I could see. It looked dark and murky to me and I couldn't see anything. He ducked my head into the water three times. The water was clean and I felt refreshed. He asked me if I could see now and I said no. He said "You can see, you just have to believe it." He took me to the edge of an abyss and asked me if I was ready to jump. I jumped and could feel myself falling deeper and deeper. It felt like I was breaking through water when I landed into a place of moving energy and colors and I moved with it. I felt that there had been a lot of work done on my fourth, fifth, and sixth light wheels (heart, throat, and third-eye chakras) and I felt a great sense of expansion and freedom.*

## Water and the Pool of Reflection

Mary Teresa's account hints at the watery nature of Dog Rose. For her, the water has a cleansing effect and provides a means of self-reflection. Jenny's experience also took her to a pool of reflection:

*In the journey to the Dog Rose, she came as a tall woman dressed in pale pink. She had stems and leaves tattooed on her arms and feet and there was a pink and green haze around her. She took me to a still pool of water and told me to look at my reflection. The water looked like silver glass. In a very gentle way she told me to "look into the water, reach deep inside yourself, and see who you really are." I could only see a vague reflection and I passed through the silver skin of the water and traveled through it, feeling like a fish. It was exhilarating and I was moving very fast. I came out*

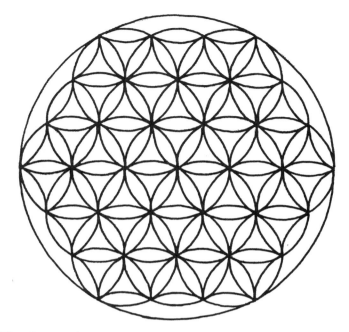

*The Flower of Life, a geometric form found in Sacred Geometry*

*in a temple with a black and white checkerboard tiled floor and intricately carved pillars. I could sense there were jaguars there although I didn't see them. I was following the scent of Roses. I climbed up three steps and found myself in front of the Dog Rose Goddess on a golden throne. There were Roses everywhere, all around her from floor to ceiling, and some of the blooms were huge with petals like dinner plates. The fragrance was extraordinary. The Goddess reminded me of Kwan Yin.\* She beckoned for me to come forward and she pressed her hand against my heart. It was electric! I gasped and it felt like I was being branded with the Dog Rose, like I belonged to her. My heart softened and began to melt and then everything melted and there was no form, only swirling colors, blues and purples, violets and pinks. The colors became fractals, spinning and pulsating, and then turned into geometric shapes. I especially remember the Flower of Life, which was lighting up with different colors in different places. There*

---

\*Kwan Yin (Guanyin) is an East Asian Goddess of Compassion.

*was also a connection with the Dog Star Sirius. It was an amazing and emotional experience and I felt the Dog Rose opened a portal to another dimension. My heart still feels physically different; it's quite tender today.*

Aoife received a graphic dream that similarly involved her own reflection, this time in mirrors:

*I dreamt I was in a hall of mirrors where a woman (an old friend who in real life I feel has betrayed me) is attacking me, trying to stab me in the back. I realize this is really self-attack. I am attacking myself and this is reflected by other people's behavior toward me. I am looking in one of the mirrors and I see myself angry, vicious, and holding a knife. I will rip my heart out. I hate myself. Suddenly I become the same as the image in the mirror and we are both angry, hating each other. We charge at each other and fight, stabbing, kicking, biting, drawing blood, stabbing at each other's hearts. We are entwined in our vicious fighting, both soaked in blood, our hearts fatally wounded, dying. Then the two images join as one being and from this bloody, gory sight two new beings arise, like two angels rising upward. These are beautiful, peaceful, loving beings; two massive angels who rise up out of the bloody mess. They embrace each other. They have such overwhelming love for each other. They come together as one being. This being becomes larger and larger. It is covering the land here [in Derrynagittah], then it is covering Ireland, then it is covering the whole of the planet. I feel I have been freed. And I feel such compassion for that poor, angry reflection. This dream makes me realize that it's time I forgave myself and others and had some compassion for myself. I think the Dog Rose is showing me how I create my own reality and teaching me about self-acceptance and compassion.*

## Learning to Say No: Compassion, Self-Acceptance, and Boundaries

Compassion and self-acceptance are recurring topics with Dog Rose. As Jenny put it, "A big theme for me was self-acceptance: This is who I am and it's okay."

Aoife continued:

*I saw how the Dog Rose can help strengthen personal boundaries. The plant is a perfect mix of openness and protection. She was teaching me how to say no to others in a compassionate way. Over the weekend I've been remembering times in my life when I've wanted to say no but I haven't. I haven't claimed my own authority and I've allowed people to walk all over me. Sometimes I just say "yes" automatically. It's such an ingrained pattern. The Dog Rose has been showing me how I really need to value and respect myself and that true compassion can mean saying no to other people as well as to my own ego.*

Linda recounted a dream with this same theme of learning to say no:

*I dreamt I was in a place with a stage and there was going to be dancing. A lot of people were around and I was up close to the stage. One man said to another man, "Ask her to dance." (The second man I know in reality. He was jailed for the rape of a woman some years back.) In the dream when he asked me to dance, I got up to dance with him. I felt I couldn't say no, even though I wanted to, because there were so many people around. I think this dream is about me learning to say no. For me dancing represents pure joy and the man in the dream represents a yucky energy, a part of myself that won't allow me to say no.*

## Dog Rose, Sound, and Transforming the Planet

Sound vibration is at the core of our reality and is a powerful transformative force. Working with sound is part of my healing practice. Sound has always been an aspect of our work in the Derrynagittah labyrinth where we incorporate various instruments including the human voice in such forms as toning, sacred chant, and singing. Toning describes a practice whereby the human voice is used to express and direct the vibration of sound. This can be done singly or in a group. During a plant initiation when our own body cells begin to vibrate with the energy of a plant, we have an opportunity to access the vibration of that plant with our voice and to direct it in a particular way. If we develop an ongoing relationship with the plant then this channel may grow. We do not necessarily tone at every plant initiation, but we have found that working with sound is particularly called for at the Dog Rose ceremonies.

Pat reported her experience. "I felt very free in my voice this weekend and really enjoyed singing. I feel it is a big part of who I am. When we were toning in the labyrinth I could see a pillar of Light and a massive Dog Rose flower over the valley."

For Sean,

> *The toning was extraordinary, otherworldly, and I felt the Dog Rose coursing through me. I saw it radiating out around us, spreading through the land, eventually throughout the whole of Ireland, and then going out through the sea, absorbing toxicity in the water and continuing to spread around the whole planet. It did a lot of cleansing and transforming of radiation at Fukushima.*

Echoing Sean's experience, Mary remarked, "The Dog Rose showed me that one way to help the Earth is to make an intention and breathe or tone it into the flowers. This way we can send it out throughout the planet." Jenny commented, "The Dog Rose was delighted we were offering a channel for its sound. The plants need channels for their gifts to come through."

## *The Goddess and the Power of the Feminine*

The Dog Rose carries a strong goddess energy that holds the power of the feminine. This common thread comes through regularly but at a recent initiation it became a potent focus for the whole group. At this particular ceremony all the participants were women, which was not deliberate and is certainly not always the case. On this occasion everyone present received a sense of the power of the feminine, which we hold within our bodies as women. Brenda gives her account of the weekend:

> *Just before the plant diet my husband Paul went into a crisis, finding it hard to breathe and his body full of tension. He was feeling very sad and*

*wondering if he had completed his mission on this planet. I would say that he has been depressed on and off over the years, but this time the grief seemed unbearable. I was not going to come this weekend but Paul pretty much insisted. He felt that coming here was the best thing I could do to help, as if he knew the Dog Rose could somehow help him. It was hard for me to leave him at home but part of me knew he was right and that it was important for me to be here. My main intention coming here was for his healing. Carole put his name on the altar and included him in the prayers and later on we sat and talked about it, which reminded me of "the talking rock" women used to gather at to discuss the problems of the community. The outcome was we started looking at how as women we can facilitate the release of grief for the men. It came as an intent to release the grief for Paul and the men of Ireland. There was something very strong in the coming together of us as a sisterhood and the power of that feminine energy. It felt like a teaching about the power that it holds. We came into the temple and holding that intention, we toned for Paul and the men of Ireland around the altar. We called to the Dog Rose and all the energies present. It was one of the most powerful and profound tonings I have ever experienced. There was, straight away, this beautiful feminine connection among the group of us and a consciousness of all the help that came in. It was so easy to access it when coming from a place of receptivity. We became this receptive bowl that was just completely filled. We had a realization that Paul was also holding so strongly for the collective and how as well as going to Paul, this was going out in a strong way to all the men. It was a very tangible bowl of energy we were working with. The Dog Rose helped bring through this power of the feminine and showed me how much beauty is there when we all support each other. It has left me with a feeling of such peace and a sense of gentle power. It has given me a glimpse of a strength and a power, on one hand feeling familiar and on another hand like nothing I have ever experienced. It gives me such a feeling of hope and really touches my heart. I am very grateful to the Dog Rose and to the community of women here this weekend.*

After returning home Brenda reported:

*When I got home I was pleased to see a big change in Paul. He was bright and cheerful, free of pain, and breathing normally. He doesn't normally say much but he described a kind of "breakthrough" point on Saturday night (the night we toned for him) and said it was the best night's sleep he'd had in ages. I felt that the Dog Rose was nurturing both of us.*

Below is an extract from a poem that came to Mary Teresa in the days following the ceremony:

> *We stood together*
> *That the male can heal,*
> *Their grief be released,*
> *And they may again feel.*
> *The love and the Beauty,*
> *The Joy and the Peace,*
> *Blessings coming together,*
> *Through gentle release.*
> *To the Dog Rose we give*
> *Our love and our thanks,*
> *To the Beings that came*
> *And led us on our Dance.*
> *The days have now passed,*
> *The ceremony done,*
> *We have gathered the blessings,*
> *Now standing as One.*

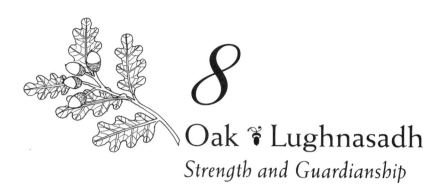

# 8
## Oak 🌰 Lughnasadh
### *Strength and Guardianship*

The mighty Oak, known as the King of the Forest, is possibly the most widely revered and loved of all our trees. The strong presence of Oak holds a central role in our consciousness. It used to be said that a person came in contact with Oak every day of his life, from newborn's cradle to old man's coffin. Such is the enduring and steadying embodiment of Oak, stretching between Heaven and Earth, holding both guardianship and protection; security and rootedness (see color plate 6). In Ireland, countless place names, including our own Derrynagittah, contain the term *derry,* which means "Oak wood"; a testimony to the abundance of Oaks that used to grow here. Still today, a few ancient Oaks stand strong in the fields and woodlands, carrying age-old memories, connecting to an ancient matrix, quietly and firmly holding their place, and contributing to the well-being of all of us.

Oaks are host to many different life forms ranging from birds and insects to plants like Mistletoe and Ivy. Of all the trees in the forest it is the Oak who supports the most creatures, reflecting the extent of Oak's generosity, strength, and ability to hold for others. Oak is ruled by Jupiter and yet it is so closely aligned to the solar cycle that some consider the sun its true ruler. Similarly, although often a symbol of kingship and thusly described as male, at other times it is held to be female and is seen to correspond to the elements

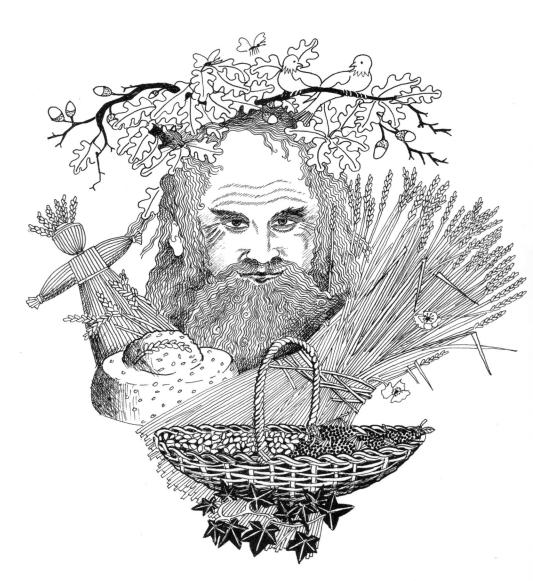

*Lughnasadh is the festival of the first harvest and celebrates the Sun God Lugh.*

of Fire and Earth. While some consider the bull to be the Oak's totem animal, this tree is also associated with stag and pig as well as a range of birds including the wren, swallow, eagle, nightjar, and woodpecker, as mentioned in various folktales from Ireland, Britain, and throughout Europe. One Irish tale tells of an Oak wood that was so fertile it drove the swine of Ireland into a frenzy. The wind would blow the scent of the Oak wood all over Ireland and wherever the scent was driven the excited pigs would rush to seek it out in droves. The colors associated with Oak are dark brown or black, and its gemstones are amethyst, moonstone, lapis, and white carnelian.

This expansive and far-reaching tree has associations with all the major Fire Festivals throughout the year. At Lughnasadh (pronounced LOO-NA-SA), as the sun's power (often considered male) begins to wane, we remember both the male and female qualities of Oak. Somewhat surprisingly, at this time of year the tree produces a new crop of fresh green shoots from the end of its branches—a sign expressing abundant celebration and making it a perfect choice for a Lughnasadh plant diet.

# LUGHNASADH
## A Time of Abundance

Lughnasadh, also known as Lammas, is the festival of the first harvest and falls around the beginning of August. This is a time of ripening and gathering. There is an abundance of food and we are beginning to gather fruits and grains. It is a time of thanksgiving and social festivities. In the past it was a time of great feasts and fairs with horse racing, games, dancing, the climbing of sacred mountains, and "doing the rounds" (prescribed sacred journeys at shrines) at holy wells. All such activities were designed to strengthen the community, the sun, and the land. Lughnasadh recalls the hero Lugh, the great Sun King and God of Light, and honors Danu the Harvest Mother. Danu is the Mother Goddess of the Tuatha De Danaan (the Tribe of the Goddess Danu) and it is she who received the finest offerings of the first fruits and grains. Croagh Patrick in County Mayo, Ireland's most famous holy mountain, is an ancient Lughnasadh site where to this day thousands make pilgrimage at the end of July.

We can celebrate the abundance of Nature by making an altar to the Harvest Mother with flowers, fruits, sheaves of grain, and home-baked bread and cakes. This can also be an excellent time to make our own pilgrimages to sacred sites. We can gather with friends around a blazing fire and give thanks for what has been our personal harvest this year. Make music, sing, and dance. Ask yourself what you fear as you go into the winter. Shout it out and give it to a stick that you offer to the fire. Rejoice in your release.

## OAK—TREE OF LIFE
*Quercus robur: Pedunculate Oak*
*Quercus petraea: Sessile Oak*
**Plant family:** Fagaceae (Beech Family).
**Other common names:** *Duir* (Irish); the Pedunculate Oak is known as the European, Common, or English Oak while the Sessile Oak is also known by the name Durmast Oak.

**Description:** The Oak grows up to 130 feet tall and can live for a thousand years. The lobed leaves are deciduous and the flowers (catkins) are borne in spring. The fruits are acorns produced in small cups.

**Habitat:** Woods; hedgerows; fields; parkland.

**Distribution:** Oaks can be found throughout the Northern Hemisphere, growing in Asia and America as far as the tropics. Europe was once covered in enormous Oak forests but now, as a result of logging, most of these are gone. The Pedunculate Oak is native to most of Europe and is abundant in Ireland and Britain. The Sessile Oak is also widespread in Europe.

**Species:** The Oak genus contains approximately six hundred species with Pedunculate and Sessile being most common in cooler regions. The Pedunculate Oak is a massive tree with a short stout trunk, wide-spreading branches, and acorns on stalks, whereas the Sessile Oak has a taller, straighter trunk and bears three to seven egg-shaped acorns in clusters directly on its twigs with no stalks. Both species can be used medicinally. North America has the largest number of Oak species with approximately ninety occurring in the United States. In North America the main species used herbally is the White Oak (*Quercus alba*). Herbalists find that Oak species may be used interchangeably.

**Parts used:** Bark (stripped from trees in the spring); young leaves (gathered in April or May); acorns (harvested in autumn); and galls—small apple-like growths formed by the tree in response to infestation by gall wasps (gathered in summer or autumn).

## Oak as a Spirit Medicine

The spirit of Oak is mighty indeed. In my early experiences with Oak medicine I was completely stunned and amazed by its sheer size, as it embodies a degree of massive physical strength that I have rarely encountered in a plant. Oak supports extraordinary stamina, tenacity, and endurance. It teaches perseverance without rigidity and that true strength comes through joy, helping people to stand strong in what may be the harshest storms of their lives. Oak gives people backbone, helping them to find the courage to be true to themselves and to move into alignment with their soul's dream. In this way, Oak can help a person to find his or her path in life. It is also eminently comforting and restorative, bringing protection, security, and groundedness. It can take someone deep within the Earth and serve as a reminder of Earth's support and at the same time it can facilitate a potent connection with the stars, planets, and all of the Cosmos. It reaches to our ancestors whether from Earth or Sky.

Oak supports leadership and integrity. It can assist at times of mental or emotional breakdown. It also helps to dissolve addictions and can give us the strength to stay present with, and to accept, the painful feelings that are at the root of addictive cravings. In Druidic tradition Oak is used magically at all major celebrations throughout the year: at Imbolc, Oak's feminine, nurturing qualities represent Brigid; at the Spring Equinox, Oak is called upon to encourage the sun's warmth; at Bealtaine, Oak is invoked for fertility; at the Summer Solstice, Oak represents the strength and glory of the sun; at Lughnasadh, Oak expresses the abundance of the first harvest by the appearance of new shoots; at the Autumn Equinox, Oak is rich with acorns and embodies the abundance of the harvest; at

Samhain, Oak comes as the unseen presence of the Sun God drawing back the veil between the worlds so that the living can reunite with the dead; at Winter Solstice, Oak is a doorway to the Light.

## Oak as a Flower Essence

**Key words to describe this essence:**
Ending struggle; accepting limitation.

Oak is one of Dr. Bach's original flower remedies, being indicated for the kind of depression and despair that can occur in usually courageous people.* The people suited to this essence often do not know when to give up or even *how* to give up. They tend to carry the burdens of others, sustaining their companions from their own reserves and ultimately becoming exhausted, depleted, discontented, and overwhelmed. Oak essence helps us to acknowledge and to accept our weaknesses or limitations. It restores hope and helps us know when to give up obstinate, relentless effort.

## Oak in Folklore and History

Oak holds a place of great importance in European mythology and there is insufficient space here to relate its innumerable myths, stories, and legends. It is one of the trees considered to be the father of mankind. The Romans believed that man sprang from Oak and the legends of many cultures refer to acorns as man's first food. The widely held sacredness of Oak has led to it being associated with a long list of deities including Zeus, Jupiter, Thor/Donar, Herne, and Thunor, all of whom rank highly in the pantheon revered by the Greeks, Romans, Celts, Druids, Anglo-Saxons, Germans, and Norsemen. In some traditions Oak was consulted as an oracular tree where the Oak oracle spoke through priestesses.

In Ireland Oak was known as one of the seven noble trees and was particularly held sacred by the Druids, who some scholars claim were known as the wise men of Oak. Irish history is full of Oaks as symbols of kingship,

---

*Dr. Edward Bach (1886–1936) was an English physician who produced flower essences in the 1930s.

the most famous being the Oak of Mugna (Moone, County Kildare). At Magh Adair (Plain of the Oaks) in County Clare there is an inauguration site where Brian Boru became leader of the Dál gCais* before going on to become High King of Ireland (inaugurated at Tara†). It is recorded that in 982, when the High King Malachy wanted to insult the Dál gCais, he cut down the sacred tree at Magh Adair. An ancient Oak known as Brian Boru's Oak still stands today in another part of County Clare near Tuamganey. It is often claimed to be the oldest Oak in Ireland. When Celtic Ireland was Christianized, the churches were sometimes built in Oak forests or under freestanding Oak trees. An example of this can be seen in the name of County Kildare (formerly *Cilldara* or *Celldara*), which literally means "the church of the Oak." It was at Kildare that St. Bridget founded a retreat called the Cell of Oak for holy women. Throughout Europe, couples were traditionally married under Oak trees long before the Christians substituted marriage in church.

Oak has traditionally been considered a gateway tree, offering a doorway to other realms. This is reflected in the Irish name *Duir,* which links with the word for "door." As an axis mundi tree, Oak represents the connection between the three shamanic realms: its roots reach down into the underworld, its trunk grows in the material plane, and its branches reach up to the heavens.‡

Oak wood is used as firewood and to make dwellings, furniture, barrels, ships, and canoes. Acorns have been food for both humans and pigs and oak bark is used for tanning leather and for making a natural purple-black dye. When gathering the leaves, wood, or acorns, it is good luck to

---

*The Dál gCais (English: Dalcassians) are a Gaelic Irish Tribe descended from Cormac Cas in the third century. They became particularly powerful during the tenth century, finally agreeing to "surrender and regrant" their kingdom to Henry VIII in the sixteenth century. Their realm was renamed County Clare. In diaspora, prominent figures from County Clare include United States presidents John F. Kennedy and Ronald Reagan, as well as French president Marshal Patrice de Mac-Mahon.

†The Hill of Tara in County Meath was the seat of the High Kings of Ireland from ancient times.

‡The axis mundi is the cosmic world axis and in many cultures this is represented by a tree, sometimes referred to as the World Tree or the Tree of Life.

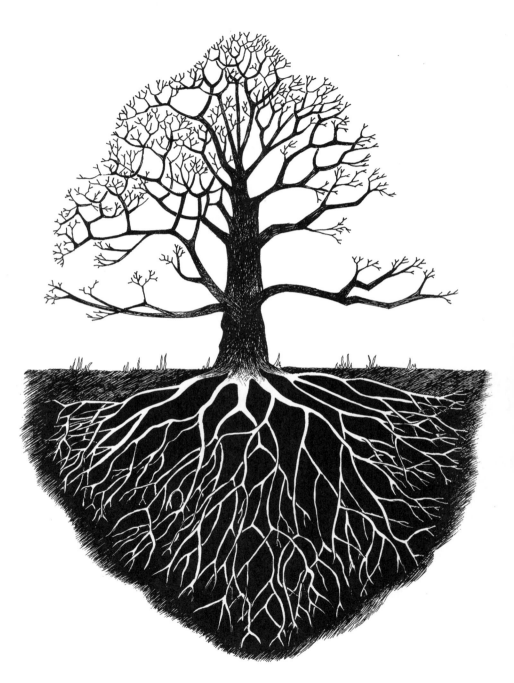

Oak is considered a World Tree linking the three shamanic realms.

feed the Oak by pouring a libation of wine on the roots. Acorns should be gathered by day and the leaves and branches by night. In Celtic lore, if it is necessary to cut down an Oak, this should never be done without explaining your actions to the tree spirit in advance and then only cut it during the waning moon. An acorn should be planted close to the old tree to provide a new home for the tree spirit.

Dreaming of an Oak tree is said to be very lucky and if acorns are growing on it, this predicts children who will make their parents proud. Reflecting its generosity of spirit, the Oak is especially well known as a tree to which humans can easily transfer diseases. This is illustrated by the following German incantation for healing gout, here translated into English: *"Oak tree, I complain to you, That the gout plagues me, I wish that it would leave me, And transfer over to you."*\* A method to help with wound healing is to take the dressing that has been on the injured body part, sprinkle it with oil of Rue, and place it inside the hollow of an old Oak. The wound will be transferred through the tree into the ground. Carrying an acorn preserves youth and brings protection, luck, and good health. Due to the deep-rootedness of Oak trees, they can be beneficial for our feet and our connection point with the Earth. Many old Oak recipes exist for ointments to heal weary feet. A decoction of Oak bark or leaves can be made into a footbath, both to soothe the feet and also to help them to find the right pathway through life. Connecting with an Oak tree and carrying one of its twigs will help bring a sense of security. Two small Oak twigs may be tied into an equal-armed cross with red cotton and carried in a pocket for protection and to aid strength and balance. Acorns are a traditional herbal treatment for alcoholism.

## Oak in Contemporary Herbal Medicine

Oak bark is extremely astringent due to its high tannin content. The young leaves, acorns, and galls are also rich in tannins and can all be used interchangeably. The astringency has a tightening and drying effect in the body. It is a tonic and antiseptic, which helps to create a barrier against

---

*Marcel De Cleene and Marie-Claire Lejeune, *Compendium of Symbolic and Ritual Plants in Europe,* vol. 1 (Ghent, Belgium: Man & Culture Publishers, 2003), 470.

infection. This makes Oak a useful remedy to tone the bowel wall in acute diarrhea when a decoction can be taken in small, frequent doses. The astringent effect can also be beneficial as part of the internal treatment of varicose veins or to dry up excessive discharges. These, for instance, can be from the digestive or reproductive systems, as in the events of colitis or noninfectious vaginal discharge. In these cases either a decoction or tincture may be taken in small, frequent doses. For vaginal discharge an Oak decoction can be used as a douche or a sitz bath by sitting wrapped in warm towels in a bidet, a large bowl, or a baby bath for twenty minutes. This same method can be helpful to heal anal fissures.

To make a decoction of the bark, small strips of young bark are boiled in water for fifteen to twenty minutes. Use ½ to 1 ounce of plant material for each pint of water. The strained preparation can also be used as a gargle or mouthwash for bleeding gums, sore throat, tonsillitis, and laryngitis. It can be made into a warm compress for hernias, inflamed glands, hemorrhoids, and sore eyes, and it can be added to a tepid footbath for chilblains or for feet that sweat excessively. Used as a lotion or compress, an Oak bark decoction makes a superb treatment for wet and weeping eczema. It dries up the fluid discharge and protects from infection. Similarly the lotion can be used to shrink varicose veins and as a wash for sores, external ulcers, and skin irritations. A compress from the decoction is particularly effective for leg ulcers that are surrounded by weeping eczema. The tannins in Oak are remarkably well tolerated by the skin and I have never seen Oak cause an allergic reaction. The decoction can also be helpful as a hair rinse to prevent hair loss and dandruff.

Ground into a fine powder in a coffee grinder, the bark can be used as a snuff to stop nosebleeds or sprinkled on a toothbrush to clean the teeth. Alternatively a naturally antiseptic and anti-inflammatory toothbrush can be fashioned from an oak twig simply by picking a small twig, chewing the end to fray it, and using this to clean the teeth and massage the gums. If you are out in nature, young oak leaves can be chewed and applied externally to bites or open wounds to ease inflammation and to promote healing. The bruised young leaves can be made into an infusion to obtain their astringent effects.

When gathering Oak bark, it should be stripped from the tree with care around the Spring Equinox, ideally before Bealtaine. Select young branches around ½ to 1 inch in diameter and use a sharp knife to cut along the length of the bark, removing small strips. The bark is fairly thick and brown on the outside and white underneath. This can be used fresh or dried in the sun or a slow oven.

## Additional Uses of Oak

The young leaves are used to make a tonic wine. Acorns are still used as pig feed and can be eaten by humans. Particularly in Germany, roasted and ground acorns are used to make a bitter tasting coffee-type drink that has nutritive properties and aids poor digestion. Some North American Oaks have more palatable acorns than those in Europe and in some forested areas of North America, acorn flour was a staple part of the diet of the indigenous people.

Oak galls (*Quercus infectoria*) or "Oak apples" are hard brown balls found on the ends of oak twigs or attached to leaves. These galls are formed by the tree's defense system in response to the gall wasp having laid her eggs in the bark of the tree. The tree uses some of its sap to produce these defensive growths. Oak galls have similar qualities to Oak bark, furthermore they are traditionally used for divination and worn for healing.

Oak wood is virtually indestructible and is a valuable construction material being durable, pliant, fine grained, and strong. Bog Oak is Oak wood that has been submerged in peat bogs for a thousand years or more. In Ireland it is frequently found in a good state of preservation and is used for sculpture making and some types of construction. In biodynamic agriculture, Oak bark is used in a preparation to rebalance the soil and protect against harmful plant diseases like fungus.*

---

*Biodynamic agriculture is a type of farming that stems from the work of Austrian philosopher Rudolf Steiner in the 1920s and advocates working with life forces, emphasizing the interaction of plants with their terrestrial and cosmic environment.

# PLANT DIETING WITH OAK

*After choosing to diet Oak, it is time to harvest the plants and prepare your elixir. Below you will find recipes for two Oak elixirs that I made at Derrynagittah. I have described the instructions that I received from Oak for making these two elixirs. When making your own elixir you will need to listen carefully to the plants and let them guide you. See chapter 4 for more complete information on harvesting plants and preparing the elixir.*

*In advance of your plant diet it is important to prepare yourself for several days with a period of physical and spiritual purification. At Derrynagittah we make specific cleansing and dietary recommendations for each diet. You will find the recommended preparations for the Oak diet below.*

## 🌿 MAKING THE OAK ELIXIR

You will notice that while most components in the elixir recipes below are expressed as parts of the whole, certain ingredients (notably vibrational essences) are listed with a specific quantity. In these cases, the amount is NOT proportional to the total amount of elixir and represents a quantity simply added to the whole. This is an intuitive, guided choice and the amount can remain the same, regardless of total quantity; that is, the same number of drops of essence can be added, whether to 20 oz. of elixir or 2 gallons.

*Elixir I*

- 4 parts Oak leaf wine
- 2 parts acorn "coffee"
- 2 parts Oak bark decoction
- 10 drops Oak flower essence

**Amount of elixir taken at diet:** Seven servings of 2 tablespoons and 2 teaspoons (40 ml) for each person

### Making the Oak Leaf Wine

For the wine, young leaves were picked in May of the previous year. It was at a time of great expansion when a planetary conjunction was occurring between the Pleiades, Jupiter, Mercury, and the sun and moon. The wine recipe is as follows:

- 1 gallon young Oak leaves
- 3.5 pounds sugar
- 1 gallon water
- Juice of 1 lemon
- Juice of 1 orange
- Juice of 1 grapefruit
- Yeast, 1 level teaspoon

Use young Oak leaves. Boil the sugar in half of the water to make a syrup; pour over the Oak leaves. Cover and leave overnight. The next day add citrus juices and yeast and pour the liquid into a fermentation jar. Add the rest of the water to make up to 1 gallon. Fit an airlock and ferment out. Rack off into clean bottles.

## Making the Acorn Coffee

Gather brown acorns in the Autumn, discarding any that are damaged. Place in a pan, cover with water, and boil for fifteen minutes. Allow to cool.

Peel off the shells and outer skins with a sharp knife. Split the acorns with a mortar and pestle and spread out to dry on a tray in a warm place for twenty-four hours.

Grind them finely and roast in an oven at 350 degrees Fahrenheit (180 degrees Celsius) until dark brown. This may take up to an hour but keep checking to avoid burning.

Use the ground and roasted nuts as you would ground coffee.

The acorns for the elixir were harvested at the end of September. Many crows were present that day. Clearly they had gathered to share the acorns and their loud cawing contributed a sense of otherworldliness. Surveying the acorns in their cups, I felt a deep ancestral bond with Oak, a presence so familiar in my life that it is like a family member who is always there, who always has been, and always will be, a part of me. I marveled at the dependable security offered by Oak, solid and secure, opening gateways to far-distant realms, and reliably holding a safe passage back.

The following spring I gathered the bark, taking small pieces from several Oaks and being careful not to take too much. Part of me dreaded this task, worried that I would damage or upset the trees. Previously I purchased dried Oak bark from my herb suppliers but this time I knew I had to strip the bark myself. In fact it was an intensely intimate experience that felt like being with a lover and even though I was already well aware of Oak's generosity, I was not prepared for the overwhelming love and joy of giving that the Oak transmitted. This experience brought me closer than ever to the spirit of Oak.

## Elixir 2

- 2 parts Oak leaves infused in white wine
- I part Oak leaf wine (see elixir I for Oak leaf wine directions)
- 3 parts Oak bark decoction
- 5 drops Oak flower essence
- 5 drops Oak gall essence

**Amount of elixir taken at diet:** Six servings of 2 tablespoons (30 ml) for each person

For this elixir I already had some remaining Oak leaf wine and dried Oak bark. In June I set out to gather additional young leaves, walking the land to connect with the Oak trees and to pay my respects. I was keenly aware of how the Oaks are holding the boundaries here and bringing protection. This day I became highly attuned to their root systems and the depth of connection they hold. I was told that at the forthcoming Oak initiation I should remind the group about our own roots, how when we are deeply grounded in the Earth we have absolutely all the support we need and we can truly reach for the skies. I was also shown how we can all be satellite dishes picking up messages, just as Oaks are. If we are grounded, clear, and properly aligned, then we can help to realign the Ancient Web in order to restore the health of the trees and to reestablish the alliance between humans, plants, and nature spirits.

## PREPARATION FOR THE OAK PLANT DIET

### General Preparations

For three days prior to diet take NO refined sugar, added salt, meat or dairy products, strong spices, coffee, alcohol, or fermented foods. Avoid oils apart from olive oil. Do not engage in sexual activity.

### Food during the Oak Diet

For those not fasting we recommend apples, hazelnuts, and honey.

### Suggested Drinks

We recommend Chamomile, Rose petal, or green tea, and hot or cold water.

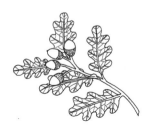

## DREAMING WITH OAK

*Through the alchemy of sacred ceremony and by surrendering to the plant, participants in a plant diet enter into an altered state in which they form close relationships with the plant that they are dieting and receive gifts that may be physical, emotional, mental, and spiritual. Many participants gain a completely new perspective on life. The relationship with the plant is deeply transformative, facilitating access to higher consciousness, guidance, and healing. In this section people who have dieted with Oak tell the stories of their personal transformations.*

## Strength of Oak

Oak initiations have proved to be eminently restorative. Not that they are easy, sometimes far from it, but always they offer a resilient strength and connection with a deep sense of peace. The strength of Oak was repeatedly referred to during these diets. Several people revealed that they had attended an Oak initiation because they felt a need for the tree's strength while others had come without expectation. Regardless, many were amazed by the strength of Oak. Participants experienced powerful feelings of awe and respect for this magnificent tree. Jenny recalled a "great sense of reverence when ingesting the plant elixir, the sacredness of taking the essence of such a powerful and beautiful being into my cells."

Ian experienced the "unending strength, generosity, and knowledge" of Oak in his description of taking the elixir. "I enjoy its sweet juices. It makes my heart shine and smile inside and out. This aroused state of awareness—the vibrational power of the Oak—is flowing through my cells, my veins. I am open and gaining its wisdom and knowledge like that of the Druids."

In addition to the Oak's strength, people frequently mentioned its peace, calmness, and patience. Linda found the Oak "so, so strong" and experienced a "deep feeling of peace and of being held." Barbara was "amazed at its rootedness and strength," while Julia said, "The Oak oozes respect and dignity."

Many initiates were able to recognize their own inner strength. After spending time with Oak, "sitting with it and being steady," Emma recalled, "I realized that I am strong. My strength is in being in touch with my emotions. I used to think that was a weakness, now I can see it's the opposite. I'm amazed. I do feel like the Oak."

Brenda attended an Oak diet during a spell of particularly stormy weather. After drinking the elixir she sat with an ancient Oak named Sirius who stands here between the labyrinth and the herb garden. Brenda gave this account:

> I went to the Sirius Oak and was invited to put my forehead against his trunk. This immediately opened up my vision and I started seeing circles and colors expanding outward. I felt a cool, sparkling blue crystal energy clearing my mind and washing it clean. It was so refreshing and I was able to just let go of all the jumble of thoughts that were going round in my head. The Oak told me to put my back against him (for me he was definitely a male) and lean on him. When I did this I felt a huge weight being lifted from my shoulders and my whole body. It was as if I had wings that were being preened and cleaned and allowed to unfurl. It was a huge relief to be with the Oak, to be unburdened and held with so much strength and comfort. The wind was so strong that I could feel the tree moving and I was amazed that he was so big and yet so flexible. I was completely connected to him as we moved together. I felt profoundly rooted and there was an incredible intimacy that took my breath away, really exciting. I realized that by connecting with him, I was connecting with all the Oaks around the world. It made my heart quicken. The wind felt fantastic and fresh, like it could blow anything away and Sirius told me that "anything is possible."

*He also said that I must learn to receive, instead of just giving, and that I am "so worthy." From the whole weekend I now have a sense of Oak as a physical body memory. I can feel Oak within me and how strong that is.*

## Stillness and Being Present

For many, the Oak's message was simple, and particularly facilitated being in the moment. Linda expressed that "Being with the Oak, it was incredibly easy to be in the present moment. I didn't have to *do* anything and it was very easy. The gift I received from the Oak was about being present and how strong and simple that is." SunSinger stated, "It kept coming down to simplicity. It's so simple. It's about coming back to that stillness," and Jane described feeling "so powerful and peaceful inside, just being."

Nicola reflected on the stillness of Oak while lying with her chosen tree:

*I could hear the birds in a faraway tree but the message from my Oak seemed to be: strength in stillness and silence. The Oak is so stable and self-assured, quietly being. I told myself to remember and absorb the Oak's strength, to be strong and self-assured. There is no need to look for affirmation from outside myself. There was a strong comforting feeling of being held by the Oak.*

The theme of self-assurance was reiterated by Maureen's experience. She imparted, "The Oak has so much security. It highlighted my insecurities and showed me my fear of not being liked by others. The message was 'Just accept yourself. It's time to be in your Power.'"

## Holding and Protection of Oak

Oak brought a deep sense of holding and protection. Jenny shared, "I am grateful for the holding. The Oak holds the space for everything to coexist. It's all held and supported. Nothing is judged. Its message was 'Trust. Be rather than do. Rest, rejoice, recuperate.'" Julia described a "strong sense of the Oak's gentle protection," reporting "the Oak helped me to open to safety. I felt held by its great and generous strength. The dream that stayed with me is one of literally being held safely and beautifully, and even play-fully, right at the top of an enormous Oak tree."

Henrique was taken back to his childhood and received teachings on the importance of holding space for himself as well as for others. He described how he had also been called to the Oak tree Sirius:

*I touched the bark and was told to "go and see my cousin" (another old Oak in a different field), "he has some stories for you." So I went to this other tree and was called to climb up it. This gave me a great sense of confidence in my physical body, trusting my body and connecting with nature, being body-free. I remembered a time when I didn't care what people thought of me. The Oak tree said his name was Rombolus. I was back in a childhood state. It opened vivid and crystal clear memories from my childhood. There was so much detail; the beautiful garden, the flowers, a tree where I used to sit and play my flute. It was pure magic. Later on in the weekend while dreaming with the Oak I found myself back in my family home before my parents' breakup. I asked to see moments that caused separation and I saw important instances of my mother and father having arguments. I was always trying to solve their problems, trying to hold space for them but completely forgetting about myself. I could not trust my father and I was trying to change him. I want to make that stop for myself and my brothers.*

### Facing Fear: Balancing Male and Female

Ciara also revisited childhood memories and described her experience of healing the masculine:

*I came here because I've been really afraid. These past few months I've been sick with fear, afraid of the dark, starting things then stopping, stuck in all aspects of my life. I feel safe here and I felt the Oak would help with fear. At first I was afraid to take the elixir, frightened to drink it. Then I couldn't get close to the tree I wanted to identify with; I was afraid to step near it. The Oak asked me, "What are you afraid of?" I said I am afraid of myself and of being seen. Fear of the masculine energy in myself. With the Oak tree helping, all of a sudden I saw myself as a big Oak tree and I was looking at myself as a little figure. I saw the Light in my heart. I was full of Light. I have huge gratitude for seeing that because now I've seen it I will never forget it, seeing myself through the eyes of the Oak. I saw the Light in my heart. I'm not judging myself so harshly now. I feel lighter. With every cup of the elixir my perception of it changed and the fear in my stomach eased. It brought up memories of childhood, of being in a hospital, and how my father was absent during important times. The masculine was absent. I went back out to the Oak and I wasn't afraid anymore. The Oak felt like the ideal male partner, like being introduced to masculine energy—real masculinity. Journeying with the Oak I realized I've been going through the Oak gateway for years; I regularly travel through the Oak. This time the Oak took me down through the Earth, past skeletons, ancestors, minerals, and accompanied by the masculine side of myself and the eagle. I met the Oak King who gave me confirmation not to be afraid. Over the weekend my dreams have been simple and with a theme of going on a journey. In each dream I meet a man and I have one of my siblings with me. It was showing me that I can have a relationship with a man without having to leave behind my siblings. The whole thing has not been easy but it was very healing. I'm not afraid now. I don't feel gripped with fear.*

Suzy experienced both male and female within the Oak. She described how she had been going through some major life changes in the past few years:

*I took a career break and went to New Zealand with my husband. I was letting go of my longing to have a child and of my longing to live outside of Ireland, and reconnecting with my husband in a different way. My life has been female dominated. There's a cold feminine energy in my family, women survivors in Belfast. They hated men; hate men. I've been looking at the part of me that hated men, that mistrusted the male inside myself. Last night it was sweet dreaming with the sacred Oak, a sacred marriage. It was very simple. I woke up and had the image of a beautiful Oak. It is man, woman, child, a divine marriage for me. I visited an amazing little oak in the winds, upright and flexible, with a very feminine energy. I wondered if I have the strength and courage to stand alone. She said, "All you need to do is trust and surrender." I asked the Oak to take away my resistances. Taking the elixir I have begun to feel the Oak in my body, sweet, long, and so sacred. I didn't have to think a thing, there was no longing, it just was. Now it feels peaceful and serene. I saw that we are all connected to the "Oak website"!*

## The Courage to Accept and Express Painful Feelings

There was no doubt that Oak touched our hearts and helped us to open to healing. Pat described how "it feels like my heart is much bigger. The Oak has really touched my heart," and Ian stated, "It really opened my heart." At one Oak diet we worked with footbaths, soaking our feet in a decoction of the bark. For Nicola, the footbath helped her to process "a lot of things relating to love in all its forms. I felt the Oak was allowing me to process and settle. I asked for, and experienced, a powerful heart healing and the dreaming allowed processing of healing the wounded heart."

For Brenda the footbath brought a lot of grief to the surface:

*I realized how desperately sad I feel about a recent relationship breakup. The Oak strengthened my heart and made it possible for me to feel the pain. I realized that I can feel this sadness and survive. I asked the Oak what is the lesson, and what came was not to blame myself. To accept that these things happen; people can be cruel. It's fine. Don't attach to it. I am okay and I have done my best.*

Emer felt that the Oak was doing heart work. She described how Oak helped her to speak the pain in her heart:

*I'm working with a lot of emotions. My mum died two months ago. I'm working with being grown up and having nobody to disappoint. When Ciara talked about her dad and the masculine it felt like a dagger. The father of my children has left and is now outside of the family. Oak gave me the realization that I haven't let him go, neither him nor my dream of us being a family. I'm saying all this so I can move on. Nobody is going to learn anything until they feel the pain and there is so much unresolved pain in families. By speaking this, the Oak can truly work for me. It is heart work, allowing people to speak their pain, healing families.*

## Allowing Ourselves to Feel the Pain of the World

In a firm and loving manner, the Oak helped us to honor our pain rather than deny it, relating both to collective issues as well as to personal well-being. Maureen expressed, "I realized I need to face the painful truth of what is happening in the world. The Oak gave me the courage to step out of the numbness and feel the intensity of the pain, not to get lost in despair but to give importance to the feelings and to let the pain move me forward into action." For Camilla, the Oak initiation brought up intense feelings of grief about trees and the Earth. She recalled how a big tree on her land had come down in a recent storm and this "shook something in me." While journeying with the Oak she was visited by Merlin and heard a voice inside of her; a warning about how "The storms are very unusual and it's a global process. We're all not on our own here anymore." She described finding solidarity with Oak and remembered how "Oak forests have been massacred all over the world," claiming, "as a nation we have almost forgotten about our Oaks." She described a "huge sadness coming through. It feels like a fracture in the right side of my body." For her, it raised the question, "Do I continue to do my little work or is there something more?"

## Interconnectedness: Balancing Heaven and Earth

Oak was commonly experienced as "a connector between Earth and Sky" as well as to the trees around the planet. SunSinger shared "a vision of all the Oak trees connecting between Russia and America. The Oaks are connecting their branches like a grid." Brenda described it this way:

*A beautiful balance of Earth being brought to Heaven and Heaven coming down to Earth, a symbiotic union. The Oak's upper branches are like a massive dish collecting and sending energy and messages from above and the enormous roots are connecting and communicating with all the roots around the planet and roots in many other dimensions too. It's like an amazing electrical network. I see it like neurons firing, and the more we humans do to reestablish a healthy relationship with the trees, the better the network functions and the more we can help the Earth come back into balance. It's actually very simple and we can really make a difference. For instance the network has been charged up by this weekend.*

Ian received "the realization of connectedness, wholeness, and One-ness with everything and everyone" while Nicola gave an account of a dream, which for her illustrated how the Oak strengthened her links with "tribe, with children, and with nature." She recalled:

*I was in an Alaska-type forest, lying by a mossy Oak tree. I walked through the door and was greeted with night fire lanterns and a forest of animals and faeries who took me through the forest on a dance/parade singing and dancing. Then the dream skipped to a big parade through the streets of Dublin co-created by a team like eco-UNESCO, kids and floats, all to raise awareness around the interconnectedness of all ecosystems on Earth.\* I heard bees (beehive floats) teaching about the soul purpose of bees. It was creating a new paradigm of a Universe where all respect the natural world; working with music, joy, art, culture, shifting the consciousness of an entire city, reaching a huge number of people.*

The following is an extract from one of my dreams that depicted the Oak as the World Tree, stretching between Heaven and Earth:

*I was in the center of the labyrinth, being invited to a ceremony and wearing a full-length green velvet gown with flowers and ribbons wound all through my hair and clothes. I could feel the Oak within me. My sap was rising and I had a strong trunk around me and deep roots that explored the earth. Through my roots I could see shining emeralds and radiant points of Light in the deep, warm soil that was teeming with life. I noticed that all the creatures from the forest were there, encouraging me. I especially*

---

\*UNESCO stands for the United Nations Educational, Scientific, and Cultural Organization.

noticed the squirrel. And around the outside of the labyrinth were throngs of people, smiling and waving.

An ancient Grandmother is in the center of the labyrinth and she comes forward and hugs me. She has been present the whole time and reminds me of a grandmother I met in Peru. I know that I know her intimately in my deepest core and yet my mind can't come up with a name. She is shape shifting in front of me. I see the faces of many goddesses and teachers and then I am looking into my own eyes and traveling down a tunnel into space. It just goes on and on, going past stars and universes and colors and lights that I can't describe. I want to cry from sheer relief and I wonder why I didn't remember before but I know I couldn't. It's really all so easy and peaceful.

An enormous Oak rises from the center of the labyrinth and stretches to Heaven. This is the World Tree. The texture of the bark is ancient and gnarled, hard yet soft, like cork that will absorb everything, and at the same time strong as an ox that will carry and support all. And these are the deepest roots I have ever seen. I am most struck by the leaves and branches, which dance with Light. I am trying to make out if they are diamonds on the leaves when I realize they are stars. It takes my breath away. I see that the Oak offers a pathway home. It's so beautiful and so vast I cannot possibly see the top. The canopy stretches into, and is, the whole Universe.

Then I look down and see there are other plants growing with the Oak from the center of the labyrinth. It's more like a beanstalk (from the story Jack and the Beanstalk), a strong vine, climbing up to the sky. I am given information that I don't understand but that I know will unfold over time. I can see that the Oak is working together with the other plants, carrying some kind of Light energy and acting as a bridge between Heaven and Earth. The Oak offers to protect all and bring courage. Each plant has its individual role. I would love to climb this beanstalk but I know I have to stay here for now. There is work to be done.

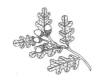

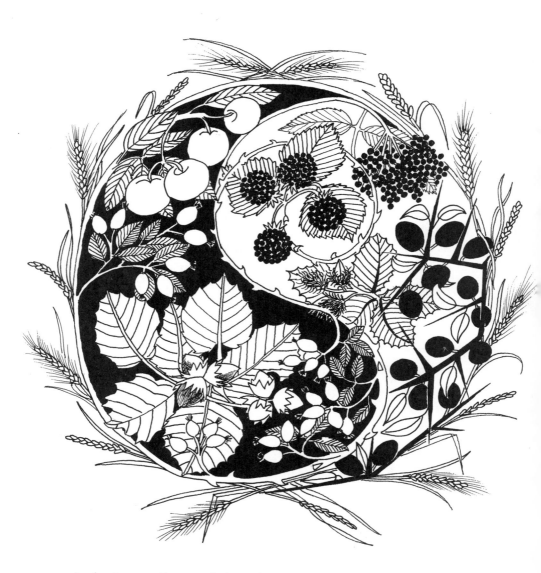

*At the Autumn Equinox light and dark stand at a balance point before the days grow shorter with the approach of winter.*

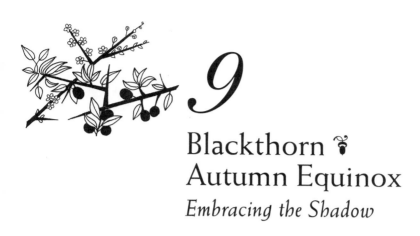

# 9

# Blackthorn ♀
# Autumn Equinox
*Embracing the Shadow*

lackthorn is a tree of transition and can be associated with a variety of points on the calendar. Blackthorn flowers are a welcome sight early in the year. Even before its own leaves are out, clouds of white blossoms light up the still cold hillsides and hedgerows (see color plate 7). Small white ball-shaped buds are interspersed with abundant clusters of star-shaped flowers, emitting an erotic, musky scent that lures insects with a promise of nectar. The pure white of the blossoms contrasts sharply with the darkness of the bark, reminiscent of light emerging from the darkness of winter, of light and dark dancing together. Considered female and linked with fierce warrior women such as the warrior queen Medb (Maeve), Blackthorn is a magical and powerful tree. The entire tree is ruled by Saturn (the fruit by Mars) and corresponds to the elements of Earth and Water. Her green, hard fruits gradually turn soft and purpley-black with a silvery-blue luster as she moves into autumn and winter, shedding her yellowed leaves and revealing her long, sharp thorns that can easily scratch and puncture the skin, causing wounds that often turn septic. Associated with goddesses of the underworld and the colors blood red and purple, her gemstones are mother of pearl and dark green malachite, while her birds are the thrush and the rook. Blackthorn has a strong and ruthless power, and demands right action. She is a much feared plant, even today. This may reflect a fear of female power, as well as the fear of our own darkness and the tendency for humans to abuse power.

Associated with spring, autumn, and winter, the magical Blackthorn can be dieted at various times throughout the year. At the Autumn Equinox, Blackthorn is in the process of transforming, standing momentarily at a balance point before going forward into the darkness of winter. She reveals her abundant harvest of purple fruits as well as her sharp thorns, which can pierce illusions and help us to look within. At this Fire Festival, as we give thanks for the harvest, dieting with Blackthorn leads us inside ourselves to transform the deepest levels of our being.

# AUTUMN EQUINOX
## *Thanksgiving and Transitions*

The Autumn Equinox, or Mabon, is a precise moment around September 20–23 when night and day are of equal length all over the world. This is the autumn harvest festival, a time to pause, to give thanks, and to welcome the coming darkness. The harvest has been gathered and all of Nature is laying up stores for the winter. Animals are storing food and some are hibernating or leaving for warmer climes. Deciduous trees are switching off chlorophyll production, revealing the red and yellow pigments beneath the green of their leaves, moving energy into their roots and transferring waste materials into their leaves to be shed and released so that they can decompose.

At this time we give thanks for the abundance of the harvest. One tradition from pagan times in Ireland is to leave gifts at outdoor shrines for the nature spirits who have helped the plants to grow throughout the summer. We can make a harvest altar with fruits, vegetables, nuts, and grains and enjoy a thanksgiving feast to celebrate all we have been given. This is a balance point, a time to pull ourselves in and bring our different aspects into balance—male and female; old and young; dark and light; conscious and unconscious. Now is a time to assess and make reparation for whatever may be out of balance in our lives. We are preparing to move toward the darkness of winter, connecting with root energy, and going within.

In Ireland numerous ancient stones are aligned with the rising or setting sun of the Autumn Equinox. On this day at Loughcrew (also known as *Sliabh na Cailli*) in County Meath, the rising sun illuminates an elaborately decorated stone at the back of one of the cairns. These solar-aligned cairns and dolmens (tombs) are mainly from Neolithic times, predating the arrival of the Celts by around two thousand years.

## BLACKTHORN—KARMIC TRANSFORMATION

*Prunus spinosa*

**Plant family:** Rosaceae (Rose Family).

**Other common names:** *An Draighnéan Donn* (Irish, pronounced UN-DRY-NON-DOWN) and *La Mere du Bois* (French for "mother of the woods"); Fruit: Sloe, Slae, Slone, Bullum.

**Description:** A dense, bushy, deciduous shrub or tree (up to thirteen feet high) with thorny angular branches and black or dark brown twigs. It bears short, lateral shoots, which turn into long sharp spines on which the flowers are borne. Often it spreads by suckering. The bark is extremely dark and on old trees becomes broken to form square plates. The leaves start off as small, pale green, and oval, later becoming longer, narrower, and dark green. A mass of pure white, five-petaled flowers appears from March to May. The fruit develops from green, unripe, and hard to a blue-black and plum-shaped "sloe," erect and containing a single seed.

**Habitat:** Blackthorn grows in hedgerows, woods, and thickets on a variety of soils (but not on acid peat) on land up to 1,300 feet in elevation. It can form an impenetrable hedge and is often found growing with Hawthorn.

**Distribution:** Widespread throughout Europe and parts of Asia, it is absent from Northern Scotland, most of Norway, and Northern Sweden. Known as "Blackthorn Plum," it is locally naturalized in eastern and northwest North America.

**Related species:** The sloe is the ancestor of our cultivated Plum. Damsons and Greengages are related species.

**Parts used:** Flowers (gathered in bud or just as they open), fruits (both ripe and unripe for different purposes; ripe fruits only sweeten after the first frost), leaves (harvested in spring or early summer), and bark (gathered in spring).

## Blackthorn as a Spirit Medicine

The spirit of Blackthorn offers strong medicine that is not for the faint hearted. This plant is very thorough and goes extremely deep. If she comes to you it is an opportunity for complete transformation, particularly dealing with karmic issues. This can be intense to say the least; it may feel severe and as if you have no choice in the matter. Take heart and remember that she can help you transform karma and live your soul's dream.

Blackthorn can bring profound emotional and spiritual cleansing, breaking through blockages, and force us to go deeper and deeper within ourselves. She is a guide in the darkness of our own underworld. One of her primary gifts is in helping us to face ourselves, to clearly see our old outworn beliefs and patterns, difficult emotions, and painful memories in order to release them. She helps us to embrace our shadow side, to recognize the capacity of our negativity, and to accept ourselves as we really are, "warts and all."

Here we are assisted in facing challenging situations with others; urged to stand in our power and authority with ruthless impeccability. When Blackthorn appears it can mean that it is time to complete unfinished business and to meet a challenge head on without backing away. She can help us stand up for our rights and demand karmic justice. We have to take responsibility for our lives and our actions and accept the consequences.

Learning about power is a major teaching here, not to use power over others but to find personal empowerment. Furthermore, the strength of Blackthorn can give support to bring out leadership qualities. Sometimes Blackthorn comes to exalt and uplift the spirit, opening us up to the healing energies of Nature and helping us to face life itself, to lift depression, and to bring hope and vitality. Protection is another major aspect of Blackthorn's spirit medicine. She is one of the most protective of plants and can form impassable barriers. She helps us to have strong boundaries and also to respect the boundaries of others.

Blackthorn is connected to all aspects of the Goddess. As mentioned above, she is associated with a range of festivals including the Spring Equinox, Bealtaine, Autumn Equinox, Samhain, and Winter Solstice.

## Blackthorn as a Flower Essence

**Key words to describe this essence:**
Facing and transforming the shadow; protection.

Blackthorn is for cutting through, helping us to pierce those things that hold us back, to purify and clear the way so we can see the path ahead of us. It assists our abilities to see our inner realities with strength and precision; transforming anger, fear, darkness, and negativity into a positive way forward. This essence carries wisdom and teaches about protection, boundaries, and invisibility (or how to pass unseen when required).

## Blackthorn in Folklore and History

Blackthorn has an ambiguous reputation, on the one hand helpful and strongly protective, on the other fierce and malevolent. In folklore Blackthorn is a tree of witchcraft and witches traditionally carry blackthorn walking sticks. These are variously described either in glowing terms as being used for protection or they are being pointed at a victim to blast the unfortunate person with a curse.

In the time of the witch hunts, numerous negative stories grew up around Blackthorn. People were accused of using Blackthorn wands with fixed thorns on their ends and carved blackthorn sticks called "black rods," which were thought to cause miscarriages and harm to others. The devil himself was rumored to prick the fingers of his initiates with thorns, with the result that many so-called witches were searched for the "devil's mark." Eventually this became the label for any mark found on the body of a suspected person and was enough to warrant a death sentence. When condemned individuals were burned, Blackthorn sticks were often used as the wood for the pyre, meant to deliver a final insult to the victim.

The story of Sleeping Beauty is just one of many fairytales illustrating how the black witch stories moved into popular consciousness. The beautiful maiden is set up by a jealous witch to prick her finger and fall into a deep sleep, thought to be dead. The maiden ends up fenced in by an impenetrable thorny thicket and the whole country is under the witch's spell until a handsome prince brings her back with a kiss. The power of love is seen to triumph over evil.

Witches aside, countless stories from Europe describe the negative use and connotations of Blackthorn. Legend tells us the thorns were tipped with poison and used to kill enemies, being called the "pin of slumber." In England it is said that Blackthorn spines were placed under the saddles of horses to make them unseat their riders when the spine went into the horse's flesh. Thorns of the Blackthorn were used for cursing by pricking wax images and in some magical traditions the Blackthorn is called the "tree of cursing." In the Tree Ogham (an ancient Celtic language where each letter is named after a tree), Blackthorn is *straif,* which many translate as "strife." Furthermore, the words *slay* and *sloe* are closely linked. In ancient Ireland a woman with no one to vouch for her was forced to clear her name by rubbing her tongue on a red-hot adze* of bronze or melted lead that had been heated in a fire of blackthorn or rowan. Today in Ireland it is still considered unlucky to bring Blackthorn into the house and some folktales say that Christ's crown of thorns was made from Blackthorn.

The Irish *shillelagh* (a club or cudgel) is made from dense, heavy Blackthorn wood and legends speak of giants who carried similar weapons. In one Irish tale, Blackthorn protects the heroes from giants and enables them to escape. They are given a twig of magical Blackthorn, which when thrown between themselves and a chasing giant, quickly takes root and becomes a whole wood of Blackthorn trees, forming a thick, tangled shield through which the giants cannot pass.

Blackthorn can also be an instrument of blessing. In previous times

---

*An ancient type of cutting tool.

in England on New Year's morning a crown or wreath of Blackthorn and Mistletoe was hung up to bring good luck for the coming year. Blackthorn crowns were burned on the fire and their ashes were scattered over the land to bless and fertilize the fields.

Traditionally Blackthorn and Hawthorn are regarded as sisters, frequently growing together and both being loved by the faeries. They were used jointly in fertility celebrations, particularly associated with erotic festivities where fertility was evoked. Blackthorn's pure white blossoms are seen as a symbol of female beauty. At Bealtaine, Blackthorn was placed on top of the Maypole, entwined in a Hawthorn garland and called "Mother of the Woods." She was also linked to Spring Equinox celebrations around the time when her blossoms appear. However, her strongest connection is with the Autumn Equinox and Samhain when her bitter fruits ripen and she is called upon for assistance with moving into the darkness and going within. At the Winter Solstice, Blackthorn wood is given as an offering to the underworld powers for the return of the sun.

## Blackthorn in Contemporary Herbal Medicine

An infusion of Blackthorn flowers cleanses the blood and is a diuretic and gentle laxative. The tea makes a useful treatment for acne and is also used as a "spring cure" (or spring cleanse) along with the unripe fruits and leaves. For spring cleansing a decoction is made from the leaves and unripe fruits, to which an infusion of leaves is added. Finally, flowers are included, soaking them in the mixture for five minutes. This is particularly beneficial for teenage boys with acne.

Most commonly used are the ripe fruits, harvested after the first frost when they have lost their bitterness. These are made into an antirheumatic syrup, which activates the metabolism and enhances general resistance, thereby also proving beneficial in the treatment or prevention of colds and flu. The pleasant tasting syrup can be helpful to flavor and enhance other less agreeable herbal medicines. Leaves are astringent and diuretic and can be used with either flowers or bark. Blackthorn bark helps to bring down fevers and is highly astringent. Unripe fruits are strongly purgative.

In anthroposophical medicine, Blackthorn extract is prepared from the flowers and considered to be particularly rich in warmth and nourishment, expressing the sun's movement and light. Rudolph Steiner recommended Blackthorn in asthma treatments and rated it highly as a strengthening and protective tonic. The plant is viewed as a preeminent strengthener, aiding general health and well-being, and is especially suitable for patients who are exhausted or drained of vitality.

### Additional Uses of Blackthorn

Sloes have long been used in wine making and to flavor gin, port, and various liqueurs. Sloe gin is still a popular drink, traditionally made by gathering sloes in late September or October, pricking them with a skewer or cocktail stick, half filling a bottle with them, adding a few spoonfuls of sugar, and covering with gin. The deep-red, almond-flavored liqueur will be ready to drink by the Winter Solstice, although it improves with age. The remaining gin-soaked sloes can be eaten as they are or processed, for instance by dipping them in melted chocolate, which is then allowed to set. The fruits also make a red dye and have been used in jam-making.

Blackthorn is a useful hedging plant for farmers. Due to the strength and density of the wood, it has been used for weapons, protective clubs, and in turnery, a form of woodworking where wooden objects are fashioned on a lathe. It also provided the teeth of hay rakes and makes the most beautiful walking sticks, revealing a rich shine when polished.

## PLANT DIETING WITH BLACKTHORN

*After choosing to diet Blackthorn, it is time to harvest the plants and prepare your elixir. Below you will find recipes for two Blackthorn elixirs that I made at Derrynagittah. I have described the instructions that I received from Blackthorn for making these two elixirs. When making your own elixir you will need to listen carefully to the plants and let them guide you. See chapter 4 for more complete information on harvesting plants and preparing the elixir.*

*In advance of your plant diet it is important to prepare yourself for several days with a period of physical and spiritual purification. At Derrynagittah we make specific cleansing and dietary recommendations for each diet. You will find the recommended preparations for the Blackthorn diet below.*

## 🌿 MAKING THE BLACKTHORN ELIXIR

You will notice that while most components in the elixir recipes below are expressed as parts of the whole, certain ingredients (notably vibrational essences) are listed with a specific quantity. In these cases, the amount is NOT proportional to the total amount of elixir and represents a quantity simply added to the whole. This is an intuitive, guided choice and the amount can remain the same, regardless of total quantity; that is, the same number of drops of essence can be added, whether to 20 oz. of elixir or 2 gallons.

*Elixir I*
- ❧ 2 parts Blackthorn flowers tinctured in gin
- ❧ 3 parts sloe syrup
- ❧ 2 parts decoction of sloes with twigs, leaves, and thorns
- ❧ 3 drops each of Blackthorn and Morgan le Fay flower essences*

**Amount of elixir taken at diet:** Seven servings of 2 tablespoons and 2 teaspoons (40 ml) for each person

Here in the west of Ireland Blackthorn usually blooms in even the coldest and wildest March weather, but the year I made this elixir we had experienced an especially long and hard winter. The Blackthorn blossoms didn't arrive until late April and early May, around a month later than usual. It had seemed like spring would never come and the early flowering Blackthorn was sorely missed. While normally I am picking Hawthorn blossoms at Bealtaine, this particular year I was harvesting Blackthorn flowers, which decorated our May altar. We also tinctured them in gin and set it aside for this elixir. Walking among the clouds of white blossoms was an inspiration reminding me that all things must change and will come to those who wait.

The sloe syrup had been prepared the previous year from sloes picked just prior to Samhain. This year, in the days before the Autumn Equinox and leading

---

*Both of these are vibrational essences made by me as part of the Derrynagittah essence range.

up to the planned Blackthorn initiation, an early frost came and the Blackthorns on the land were calling out to be included in the ceremony. Therefore, with the addition of various other plant parts, I harvested sloes to make a decoction. The additional parts included three twigs, three leaves, and three long, rigid blackthorn spikes. After straining the decoction it was ceremonially combined with the other ingredients, including essences of Blackthorn and Morgan le Fay. I had strongly felt the spiritual presence of Morgan le Fay while picking the sloes and this was powerfully reinforced during the making of the elixir. Commonly known as the half-sister of King Arthur of England, Morgan le Fay is one of the most misunderstood of the Celtic deities. Known as the "Divine Drop" or the essence of the Holy Grail, her being encompasses both human and angelic consciousness. She is a warrior goddess, famed for her ancient wisdom and healing magic, including a deep knowledge of healing plants. The Morgan le Fay essence connects with her energy and carries the attributes described below.

> **Key words to describe this essence:**
> Magic; freedom; faery magic; mystic marriage; oneness.

Morgan le Fay essence is made from Herb Robert and Black Knapweed. It connects with Morgan le Fay, frees the magic of the land and the magic within us, bringing freedom for the enchantress and the enchanted. This essence awakens faery magic and carries the alchemy of Fire and Water. It helps the creation of the Rainbow Bridge that leads to the mystic marriage and the remembrance of Heaven and Earth as One.

### Elixir 2

- ❧ 3 parts Blackthorn decoction (made from simmering leaves for twenty minutes and then adding flowers and buds, leaving them to soak for five minutes). This liquid was cooled and strained, then preserved by adding gin (30 percent by volume).
- ❧ 2 parts Blackthorn elixir from a previous diet
- ❧ 4 parts sloe gin
- ❧ 7 drops Blackthorn flower essence

**Amount of elixir taken at diet:** Six servings of 2 tablespoons (30 ml) for each person

For this elixir the Blackthorn buds, flowers, and leaves were picked and prepared in March around the Spring Equinox. During the harvesting, my overwhelming feeling was one of gratitude. I experienced a huge outpouring of love from my heart and gave thanks to the Blackthorn for her many generous gifts. I felt a strong connection with the stars as well as with the Primroses who were just beginning to flower. Some of the Primroses wanted to be picked and included, claiming that they would enhance the Blackthorn elixir. I was not convinced of this, feeling that they were having a game with me and seeking attention. While sometimes additional plants can be entirely complementary, this is not always the case and when harvesting it is important to have focus and discernment to avoid distractions! The sloe gin was prepared the previous winter from sloes picked after the first frosts.

## PREPARATION FOR THE BLACKTHORN PLANT DIET

### General Preparations

For three days prior to the diet take NO refined sugar, added salt, meat or dairy products, strong spices, coffee, alcohol, or fermented foods. Avoid oils apart from olive oil. Do not engage in sexual activity.

### Food during the Blackthorn Diet

For those not fasting we recommend apples, pears, plums, almonds, honey.

### Suggested Drinks

We recommend Chamomile, Lavender, or green tea, and hot or cold water.

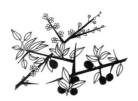

# DREAMING WITH BLACKTHORN

*Through the alchemy of sacred ceremony and by surrendering to the plant, participants in a plant diet enter into an altered state in which they form close relationships with the plant that they are dieting and receive gifts that may be physical, emotional, mental, and spiritual. Many participants gain a completely new perspective on life. The relationship with the plant is deeply transformative, facilitating access to higher consciousness, guidance, and healing. In this section people who have dieted with Blackthorn tell the stories of their personal transformations.*

## Fear of the Unknown, Physical Effects, and Getting Well

The Blackthorn elixirs have tended to have a popular taste, being described as "beautiful like gold" and "nectar from heaven." For Grace, the pleasant flavor was unexpected and highlighted her fear of the unknown:

> I am used to taking plant medicine and I was expecting something rotten. I was very surprised that it was so delicious. In my nature I am always cautious of the unknown. I always do things, but I come with a holding back of myself. The Blackthorn taught me that there is unexpected sweetness in the unknown as well as fear. To have the experience of the sweetness has made me really trusting.

Sometimes taking part in a plant initiation causes physical vomiting as an aspect of purification, traditionally described as "getting well." In this example, Grace recalls how she underwent an immediate physical cleansing after drinking the elixir. "It went into my system really quickly and I was in an altered state of consciousness and sick from the start. It has affected my body, wiped out everything in my head, eyes, and ears. During the first night and all the next morning I was physically sick."

Joan experienced a strong physical reaction after meeting the Blackthorn tree:

> I met the Blackthorn beside the herb garden. That just wiped me out altogether. When I met the tree and touched her leaves it was like meeting an old friend, very emotional—it was so compassionate and loving. I was shocked to realize that I had forgotten the love and understanding we had for each other. When I came back to the temple my body was really aching and I got a bad pain in my head. I didn't know if I would make it into

*the temple. I don't remember a lot of what happened after that. What came was the amount of abuse both women and Blackthorn have suffered. The Blackthorn was used by men to kill women and I felt the horror the Blackthorn also felt in this. It was like women and Blackthorn were one and the Blackthorn was in shock for being used to beat women to death. There was great love from the Blackthorn. This is what went on for me for the duration.*

Reflecting afterward, Joan commented:

*It was about a past life when I was beaten to death because I didn't conform and I had a belief system that was outside Catholicism. It feels to me that a lot of the pain I experienced at the plant diet was about restriction. How when you get caught in one belief system you can lose your heart and there's no give, no seeing other people's points of view. Living in that rigidity causes a lot of pain and at the time I was living in rigidity. Since the experience with the Blackthorn I am seeing my rigid beliefs more clearly and I can be more compassionate.*

## Offering a Group Blessing

A common practice at our ceremonies is to offer a group blessing for the plant being dieted. We visit one or a group of the plants growing on the land, speak our blessings in turn, and leave our gifts. In this instance we visited three Blackthorns that grow together by the riverbank and are seen to represent the three aspects of the triple Goddess, the maiden, mother, and crone. For many participants, offering blessings to Blackthorn was particularly memorable. Pat recounted, "The blessing ceremony was just wonderful by the river and people's honoring and love for the trees was very moving." She continues, "I had a sense that the plant wanted to be redeemed. It wanted us to realize what we had done to her in the past and she wanted to be honored for her gifts. She said she would like respect and remembrance from me."

Brenda described a similar experience, including her perception of the Blackthorn's gifts:

*The blessing at the river I found really moving, both in hearing people's appreciation of the trees and Nature and observing the response of the Blackthorns, which was beautiful. They were responding differently to each person. With one person, when she stood in the middle of the three trees they all linked together and put their arms around her. For everyone the Blackthorns gave so much and it felt so good to be honoring Blackthorn when it has been so badly treated in the past.*

## *Joy, Ease, Lightness, and Beauty*

Despite the Blackthorn's fierce reputation, an overwhelming number of participants described experiences and messages of joy, ease, lightness, and beauty. Joan, while feeling extremely heavy, was told to "Lighten up." Grainne received the advice to "choose the easy" and to "laugh your fears and sorrows away." Mary recalled, "the diet was very easy, smooth, and loving."

Linda was inspired to walk the labyrinth with the intention "to reclaim joy, to really live life with absolute joy." She felt Blackthorn was working through the family dogs, as she put it, "Before I left the Labyrinth both dogs were trying to sit on my lap and lick my face, trying to say 'it is this easy.'" Angie also received a message about how to live her life, explaining, "It is about doing what is joyful for me and expressing my joy."

Pat was reminded that growing old can be joyful. She recounts, "I felt the crone tree wanted to say something to me. I felt what she was saying was that old age doesn't have to be infirm. At times I get scared that I will get more and more infirm and the tree said that old age is not a ponderous thing; it is joyous and agile." This transformation of fears is a common theme that we will return to later.

Grace emphasized the beauty she experienced. She described the feeling of coming home and the connections with her mother who had recently passed away:

*When we went onto the land and into the herb garden it was so beautiful. It is like the whole weekend has been such a pleasure and beauty is the only word. The night was spectacular—holding the real beauty of the plants and the beauty of the skies and heavens. At the same time I was really sick and with the sickness came negativity, so holding all of that together and being able to hold it and see it clearly. It was fabulous. It felt like coming home to myself. It had a lot to do with my mother whose whole life was spent with plants and she was deeply connected with sacred sites and the Hawthorn, which is like a sister to the Blackthorn. So connecting with the Blackthorn was like connecting with her in a different way and making a new relationship with my mother.*

Anna shared that Blackthorn brought her the gift of creating love and beauty in her life. She remarked, "This is a gift I am searching for and the world is waiting for."

## An Inspiration of Music and Dancing

As well as encouraging joy and beauty, Blackthorn inspired and uplifted us with music and dancing. Music is always a feature of our ceremonies but was overwhelmingly strong with the Blackthorn, ranging from our own singing, chanting, and didgeridoo playing to the ever-present bird song. While out on the land and commonly accompanied by a host of birds (robin, blackbird, and crow to name a few), many of us were called to play different notes on the thorns themselves and Brenda was instructed to make a rainstick (an instrument that makes the sound of falling rain) using Blackthorn spikes.

Angie realized how much she was missing music in her life:

*The Abba song "Thank You for the Music" came to me and this has been a bit of a thing going on all weekend—that I don't have very much music in my life. It seems that music is really important to me and I need to bring it more into my life. I had a dream that was about my partner and myself and how we have had a good time together. So that was lovely. Now I realize that my partner is a musician and my whole life could be filled with music, but I have been shutting it out.*

Our dancing was described as feeling "like a party, a perfect celebration of something very new. It was an amazing way to embody the plant, to really feel being seed, root, flower, leaf, sloe, everything." Like many others, Linda shared that she "loved the dancing" saying, "I know it is a way through for me." Pat had been concerned that dancing would aggravate an old pain in her knees, absent since an earlier plant initiation. She shared, "This time I felt what was holding me back was just fear. When I was dancing my knees didn't hurt at all. At the end I felt very young, very open, and very clear. The dancing was fantastic. I woke up this morning feeling amazing."

Angie recalled, "It was lovely to move and to dance with Blackthorn. It was just gorgeous." She received the message "to let go of the ego, that is the beauty," and revealed "when I let go of my self-consciousness it is deeply healing for me to move." Brenda found that dancing with Blackthorn brought about a release of grief. "I felt lots of Blackthorn spikes going into my throat and releasing a load of grief. At the end of the dancing the spikes came again and pierced it all, which transformed it in a kind of purple haze. There was also the grief of the Blackthorn being released."

## Clearing Old Patterns and Transforming Fear

The letting go of old patterns and emotions is a strong theme. Angie went on to describe her experience with the GreenBreath during which a powerful release occurred:

> I had one of the most profound experiences of my life. It was really overwhelming. When [Carole] spoke about the ancestors I felt a strong connection with that. It was great for me to make a noise as I often hold back and don't make any sound. Toward the end it was very peculiar. All I am conscious of is that my hands just tightened into fists and I was really rigid. I couldn't open out my hands until we had finished and the pain felt like I couldn't bear it. I felt it was a tremendous gift and I don't know what I was shedding but I felt that it was time and I am delighted to have gone through that. It feels like it has opened the way forward and maybe I have some gift in my hands.

Linda revealed that she had resistance to doing the GreenBreath saying, "I decided to go for it and every time I came to a block I would ask the Blackthorn to cut through it for me. I felt in the end that there was a big release." My own experience, while facilitating the GreenBreath and observing the group, was of Blackthorn spikes coming in and piercing different things for different people, like hammering in different nails and releasing an enormous amount of toxicity.

Terri gave her account:

> I was panicking in the GreenBreath because I felt I couldn't get my breath and I know that fear is blocking me because I fear for the planet and for my children's future. I decided to let it go and I thought of other things to let go of, like jealousy and regret. Moving to the music was very cathartic and allowing the Blackthorn to cleanse each chakra and making a rainbow bridge to the tree was very powerful. I became the Blackthorn and then I knew that I was also part of Nature and not separate from it. It was a revelation of joy and a very ecstatic experience. I thought I was going to float away off the floor. I never felt so relaxed in my life. Back at the labyrinth I came to know what I have to do and it is all about trust.

## Releasing Karma and the Right Use of Power

Later on, while dreaming with Blackthorn, Bridget met with the Guardians of Karma whom she had decided to call upon for karmic release:*

> When I enter they are waiting for me and I ask to release the block held in my throat. First they say "no" and show me two past lives (one with a rope around my neck and one with hands around my neck) that I have to release first. They explain that in order to release the karma, I must be willing to correct the underlying beliefs, attitudes, and character traits that led to the karma in the first place. Otherwise I am likely to repeat

---

*The Guardians of Karma are highly evolved spiritual beings who are the supreme keepers of karma; they will sometimes grant karmic release. In our system of working with the Medicine Wheel, the Guardians of Karma are associated with the direction of the Northwest, the place of cycles and patterns, karma and dharma. The Northwest area of the Medicine Wheel herb garden houses a *souterrain* (a stone chamber) that one can enter in order to call on these beings. This is what Bridget is referring to in her story.

*the pattern and create more of the same. I tell them I am willing to correct these things. Then I go back to the original question and they say, "It is done. Believe," implying that I must trust the process and really believe it is possible. They also tell me that I still have to nourish my throat and pay attention to it, for instance by giving it herbal medicines. I must not neglect my throat. Then they give me some teachings about power and discernment, saying that I must acknowledge myself as a woman of power and it is not necessarily appropriate to share what I know with every other person. This is proper discernment and does not mean I believe myself to be superior or that I am abusing power. Actually it is the reverse. It is the correct use of power since it means I know when to reveal something and when not to, for the highest good of all. This is a surprise to me and feels like a major revelation that will change my life. I can see it is the only way I can truly embody my own power. I know this is also about boundaries and protection. They showed me when to speak and when not to speak, that sometimes it is important to know when to keep silent—when to share and when NOT to share. And I don't have to share every part of myself with others. This is a big teaching for me. I am very grateful to have been given so much.*

## Reclaiming the Power of the Feminine

Reclaiming one's power is a strong message from Blackthorn. Grainne related how the diet brought up her fear of her power as a woman while Anna reported, "the Blackthorn told me she can help me be the medicine woman that I am." Brenda received the message, "Blackthorn can help us find our way back to the ancient women's ways and the knowledge and traditions of the Grandmothers, which can help the world at this time."

The power of the feminine was strongly evoked during this encounter imparted by Erica:

*It was easy to diet with the Blackthorn; exciting and joyful too. I could hardly wait to drink the elixir and to be in the presence of the tree. I felt no fear. I wanted to be among its branches, to feel a part of it. Something in me was already in its tune. The internal pulsing I felt before had been a source of anxiety for me. It was like a dizziness in my head and I worried it would become vertigo. In my connection with Blackthorn, however, there was a rightness about it, an exact match, a fit. In a recurring dream I used to have, I was extremely concerned at having lost something very important and there was a desperate need in me to find it again. It seemed to be about a stick. Now I wonder if that was Blackthorn.*

*An Draighneán Donn (the Irish name for Blackthorn) is like a beautiful woman. I knew exactly which tree called to me and immediately I wanted to sing to her. I think she likes music and song. While I was with her, birds came to visit—a robin and a blue tit. A bee was buzzing and the wind rustled in the leaves. It was a rich sound experience. The first lines and the melody of the Irish song "An Draighneán Donn" came to me as I sat with Blackthorn:*

Síleann céad fear gur leo féin mé nuair a ólaim lionn.

*I was taken aback by this and I paused to take it in:*

A hundred men think I'm theirs when I'm drinking beer.

*Blackthorn to me is associated with reclaiming my sovereign self. It's about accepting my feminine power—receiving it, trusting it, acting on it. In the time I spent with Blackthorn, I was fully grounded, not in reverie. Ideas came to me. It was all very real.*

Reiterating the theme of empowerment, Linda described how she was urged to stand in her power and speak out for what she believed in. She recalled, "In taking the drink, the Blackthorn felt incredibly strong and like a real warrior energy. For me it was telling me to speak out, really urging me to say what I felt strongly about."

Linda went on to explain how Blackthorn encouraged her to stand as a warrior for the land, and how this related to her desire to keep Ireland free from fracking.* She described her recent visit to County Leitrim:

---

*Fracking is hydraulic fracturing in which water, chemicals, and sand are pumped down deep wells under high pressure to break up rock and release natural gas, which can then be used for fuel.

*I decided to go on a bit of a scout to find out about fracking and see what was happening there. It was very interesting, but it is all a bit sinister in that one of the people I spoke to told me that all the rights for the gas underground have been already sold. The IMF (International Monetary Fund) is putting pressure on the government to use every resource to pay back their debt. I can't be apathetic and expect everything to be okay. I had this really strong feeling of us standing together as a people and saying that we are not going to take this. What came at the end of the Blackthorn journey was that we have to try to do things ourselves to stop fracking. The message from the Blackthorn was that I have to stand for the land and stand for the Earth. I have to use my warrior energy. I asked the Blackthorn for the gift of courage and I made a commitment to stand for the land.*

## Making a Commitment

Blackthorn seems to call for, and inspire, commitment. At one of the Blackthorn initiations the entire group decided to pledge their commitment to unity consciousness by committing to consistently follow divine guidance rather than our egos.

Terri expressed how

*The Blackthorn wants us to put our heart into everything and nurture with our heart power. From this weekend I've learned that the Blackthorn gives the power to put your heart into things but it protects you at the same time. You can put your heart into something but remain detached as well. When I was with the Blackthorn I got an impression of a woman of uncertain age. She had a green dress on and she had leaves and fruit on her neck and a garland of flowers in her hair. She wanted to run through the woods. She made me feel very comfortable and safe and she gave me the message "Trust in your own ability to trust and allow inner guidance to come."*

Afterward she described how

*On the way home a fox appeared and crossed the road in front of us. For
me, the fox brings the message to "trust wholly and fully in yourself and in
your abilities. Your gift is to have a creative mind. Do not doubt yourself or
your path." I thought that was amazing given that trust was such an issue
during the weekend and was one of the gifts of the Blackthorn.*

## *Freedom and a New Beginning*

Others reported feeling "liberated by the Blackthorn" and "freed from
some very old karmic patterns." Bridget experienced a "complete new
beginning," and Anna related, "I think I have a very strong connection
now with the Blackthorn. I have her inside me and when I need them to,
the thorns can sprout out. The commitments felt very sacred and important to do. I feel I must remember them."

The final words here are from Grace: "The Blackthorn, I just love it,
and that tiny flower, I can't wait for it to come in springtime. It is a real
privilege to have it in my system now."

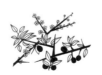

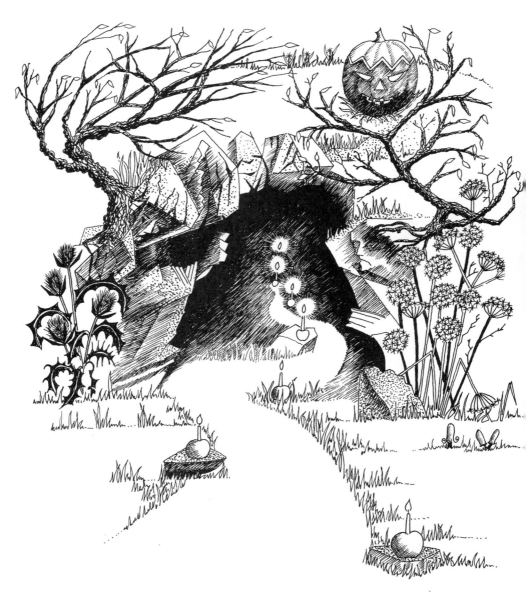

*At Samhain we honor the dead when the veil between the worlds is thin.*

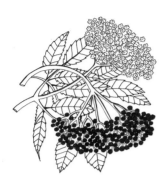

# *10*
# Elder ※ Samhain
## *Ancestral Healing*

*K*nown in many lands as the Elder Mother, Elder is an ancient faery tree connected to the crone or dark aspect of the Goddess (see color plate 8). Famous for her powerful healing abilities, she is a highly valued and respected plant, well able to speak for herself:

> *I am the Elder Mother, the ancient tree that speaks.*
> *I am the Master Herbalist, keeper of the serpent's wisdom,*
> *    holder of the cunning secrets of old.*
> *I am the Tree of Life, fixed and grounded as my roots,*
> *    reaching to the sky as my highest branches.*
> *I am the Tree of Death, the owl that flies in the darkness, the*
> *    rook that sets you free.*
> *I am the red cauldron of regeneration, the wise Crone who*
> *    sees beyond the past and reaches through the future.*
> *I am as old as old can be, carrying the wisdom of the ancient*
> *    stories, whispering on the wind.*
> *I am the fruit of the Tree of Knowledge, the seed that dwells*
> *    within, the song of the Ancient Ones.*
> *I am the dancer with Venus, the lover of beauty and the*
> *    seeker of harmony.*

*I am the tenacity and perseverance of badger; I dig deep into
the earth and I never give up.*

*I am the frothy abundance of summer blossoms; the dark,
dripping berries of autumn and the gnarled, twisted
skeleton of winter.*

*I am malachite and green jasper, my jewels shining as I bless
and welcome the faery train.*

*I am the Guardian of the Sacred, standing with ruthless
impeccability, dependable with integrity.*

*I am the magical teacher who sees all and knows when to
hold her silence.*

*I am the Elder Mother, the ancient tree that speaks.*

Intimately connected to death and rebirth, Elder is a potent tree to diet with at Samhain. Often called the witch's tree, Elder connects with ancestral energies and brings blessings of wisdom and healing, regeneration and renewal.

# SAMHAIN
## *Remembering the Dead*

Samhain (pronounced SOW-AIN) or Hallowe'en, is a crucial and transformative time of year falling around October 31. Literally the "end of summer," it marks the start of the Celtic New Year, a time of death and rebirth, of endings and beginnings. This is a magical time when the veils between the worlds are thin and there is easy communication with those who have passed over. We honor our dead ancestors and loved ones, welcoming them into our homes with prayers and offerings of food left on altars and doorsteps. As the days shorten and the dark increases we descend into the darkness and mystery of our inner selves, from which new life will ultimately arise.

This is the festival of remembrance. We remember our departed loved ones by placing their photos and mementos on the altar, always leaving a place for them at the feast. We can light a sacred fire to purify and let go, allowing parts of ourselves to die in order to be reborn. A powerful ritual is to burn an effigy made from sticks and grasses to signify all that is being released from the old year. This is also an ideal time for inner journeys and divination, a time to look into crystal balls, mirrors, or pools of water to receive guidance and to see your destiny for the coming year.

At Samhain the faery mounds are believed to open and this is the time that humans can most easily be abducted into faery realms. Beings from the otherworld emerge and are visible to humans. One such entrance to the otherworld is Oweynagat, or the Cave of the Cats, in County Roscommon, said to be the home of the Morrigan, Goddess of War and associated with Great Queen Medb (Maeve).

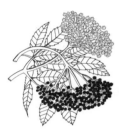

## ELDER—EARTH MAGIC
*Sambucus nigra*
**Plant family:** Caprifoliaceae (Honeysuckle Family).

**Other common names:** *Ruis* (Irish); Elder Mother; Black Elder; Witches' Tree; Judas Tree; Lady Elder; Devil's Eye; Tree of Doom; Old Lady; Whistle Tree; Pipe Tree; Dog Tree; Plant of the Blood of Man.

**Description:** A small deciduous tree or large shrub up to twenty feet tall, with arching branches and oval, pointed, finely serrated leaves. Elder bears fragrant clusters of creamy-white, five-petaled flowers in summer followed by purple-black berries in autumn. The bark is corklike and brownish grey.

**Habitat:** Woods, hedgerows, riverbanks, roadsides, and waste ground. A prolific grower, Elder sends up shoots anywhere and grows easily from cuttings.

**Distribution:** Native to Europe, Asia Minor, West Siberia, and North Africa, Elder has grown in Ireland for millions of years and is found throughout the country. Its seeds are frequently dispersed by birds that eat the ripe berries. Several closely related native species are distributed throughout much of North America and are often treated as a subspecies of *Sambucus nigra,* as in the variety *Sambucus nigra* var. *canadensis.*

**Species:** The American Elder, otherwise known as the American Black Elderberry or Sweet Elder (*Sambucus nigra* var. *canadensis*), with dark purple berries can be used interchangeably with Black Elder (*Sambucus nigra*). The North American Red Elder (*Sambucus racemosa*) with red berries should not be used. Dwarf Elder (*Sambucus ebulus*) has unpleasant smelling leaves, white (sometimes pink-tinged) flowers, and black fruits. Although not common, it can also be used.

**Parts used:** Fully open flower heads harvested in early summer and used fresh or rapidly shade dried in no more than 95 degrees Fahrenheit (35 degrees Celsius) are best. Flowers can be used for infusions or tinctures. Berries can be gathered ripe in September, separated from stalks, and used fresh or for juice. Berries can also be dried for use in decoctions, syrups, or tinctures and frozen to use at a later time. Leaves harvested in spring or summer can be used fresh or dried.

## Elder as a Spirit Medicine

As a spirit medicine, Elder brings innumerable blessings of healing, protection, and abundance. Elder may appear during healings to help people connect with their inner wisdom and to remember and value what they know inside. Elder offers quiet confidence and unshakable strength to follow one's own truth. Many times the ancestors will speak through Elder. The tree opens up vision, clears blocks in the third eye or sixth light wheel, and opens a channel of communication with the invisible realm. This can be helpful for making contact with plant spirits and faeries as well as generally enhancing clairvoyance, bringing insight and the understanding of dreams. Furthermore, Elder can be called upon to help the dead cross over.

The healing power of Elder cannot be overestimated. With remarkably gentle force, Elder carries out seemingly miraculous healings on all levels: physical, emotional, mental, and spiritual. It brings both blessings and protection and helps us to become a blessing in the world. As a blessing herb, Elder is good for blessing people, places, or things. One simple method is to scatter the leaves and berries to the four winds, in each direction visualizing and naming whatever is to be blessed. This procedure can also be used to protect you from negativity.

The bruised leaves, traditionally gathered at dawn or dusk on the last day of April, are boiled in oil. Most often linseed oil is used, but one could also use extra virgin olive oil. This *oleum viride* (green oil) is used as an anointing oil for protection, to invoke the Elder Mother, and to bring about visions of the otherworld. This oil can be particularly appropriate for use at Samhain.

## Elder as a Flower Essence

**Key words to describe this essence:**
Self-appreciation; releasing judgment; deep healing.

Elderflower essence brings appreciation for the self and the ability to see the value of all other beings. It helps us to get out of the box and no longer see life in black and white, dissolving judgment and fixed ideas. Elder can help us to travel deeply within ourselves to address profound emotional and psychological blockages. It offers deep healing and enhances past life recall.

## Elder in Folklore and History

Elder is an important ancient plant, steeped in myth and folklore. It has so many healing virtues that, as early as 400 BCE, Hippocrates described it as his "medicine chest." Dedicated to Thor the Thunder God and to Freya, Goddess of Fertility (the most revered of all goddesses in Norse mythology), over time the tree became known as the Elder Mother, or as *Hylde Moer* in Scandinavian and Danish legend. Few plants have evoked so much fear and respect. The Elder Mother is an incarnation of the old Faery Queen, the dark goddess or crone aspect of the Triple Moon Goddess. She works strong Earth magic. It was thought that when an Elder grew in your garden it meant that she had chosen to protect your house, and if you were foolish enough to cut the tree without asking permission, she might follow and plague you, as she does to any who use her with selfish intent. Certain Native American tribes believe that Elder is the mother of the human race. There is evidence that Neolithic people ate the berries and that the Ancient Egyptians used them medicinally. In parts of Europe, people would kneel down and pray before an Elder prior to pruning it and the Dutch professor of medicine Herman Boerhaave (1668–1738) was seen always to raise his hat to an Elder. Still today in some country districts of Europe, wise people show their respect by touching their hats when passing an Elder tree. A friend of mine from Switzerland has related how his father taught him that he should always raise his hat to greet an Elder and kneel down to greet a Juniper. There are long-held associations between witches and Elder. Legend has it that witches often lived in Elder trees and were able to transform into them. One story from Northamptonshire in England tells how a man who cut an Elder stick for his son was horrified to see the tree bleed. On their way home, father and son met their neighbor, a suspected witch, and noticed she had a freshly bloodstained bandage around her arm. In Ireland, Elder was used for the handles of witch's broomsticks and wreaths of Elder were woven as crowns and worn by witches at Samhain to enhance their communication with those who had crossed over. Elder is a tree of the dead and was used as the wood of the pyre at cremations. In Europe it was also commonly planted in graveyards and placed in the coffin at burials. A gateway tree, her roots were seen as the doorway to the otherworld. She was also once a feature of popular erotic love, a custom thought to arise from her blooming with the peaking of the sun's energy at the Summer Solstice.

Considering Elder's associations with female power, sex, and death, it is perhaps not surprising that she was sometimes feared. Frowned upon by the early Christian church, she was vilified and given strong negative associations. Christ was said to have been crucified on an Elder tree and Judas was thought to have hanged himself on one. A plant of the faeries and rich in magical power, superstition paired Elder with Hawthorn, their feared qualities illustrated by this old English rhyme:

*Hawthorn blossoms and elderflowers*
*Fill the house with evil powers*

Elder became known as a wicked tree and it was said that burning Elder in the fireplace might invite the devil to come and sit on the chimney, while to make a cradle of Elder wood was as good as giving the baby to the faeries!

However Elder never lost its reputation as a healer and benefactor. A popular and widely used herbal medicine, the buds, green leaves, bark, flowers, seeds, and berries were all used in some way to treat a wide range of disorders, many still popular today. In Switzerland the bark is said to be purgative if gathered by scraping downward and emetic if gathered by scraping upward. Elder's uses in magical healing were described by the Roman scholar Pliny the Elder in 77 CE and Elder has been employed for hundreds of years in a variety of magical healing applications, as well as for blessing and protection. It was a popular tree on which to transfer a whole range of illnesses, and in Germany and Denmark, as recently as 1920, it was customary to tie a strip of bandage around a branch of Elder in order to get rid of fever. In the nineteenth century the Elder was used in England, France, and Belgium to defend against sorcery, and it was believed to protect against fire and lightning and to keep eggs, milk, and butter fresh. Pungent Elder blossoms were a traditional decoration at weddings to bring good luck to the couple and in Sweden pregnant women would kiss an Elder tree to bring good fortune to an unborn child and to ensure a protected birth, while sick people would sleep in the shade of an Elder in order to be cured. Elder was known as the tree of regeneration because it illustrates the regenerative powers of life by its ability to root from any part of itself, to send up vigorous shoots from its base, and to regrow damaged branches. The Elder's hollow stem was said to have been used by Prometheus to bring fire to man from the gods, and children have long used the same stems to make simple flutes and popguns.

## Elder in Contemporary Herbal Medicine

The flowers and berries are powerfully healing and fortifying, with the blossoms being the most commonly used therapeutically. Elderflowers remove mucus from the body and make an ideal remedy for feverish colds and flu. A hot infusion stimulates the circulation and promotes sweating, thereby cleansing the body by eliminating toxins through the skin and resolving fever and infection. They are ideal for childhood fevers and can be drunk hot to induce a sweat or added to a bath or footbath. Elderflowers combine well with Peppermint and Yarrow to reduce the length and severity of colds and flu and are indicated for any catarrhal conditions of the upper respiratory tract such as sinusitis and persistent nasal congestion. The catarrhal deafness and tinnitus from mucus buildup due to inflammation of mucus membranes both respond well to Elderflowers. Combined with Nettle tops, they make an excellent remedy for hay fever and other allergic conditions, reducing mucus secretions and bringing down swelling of mucus membranes in nasal passageways and bronchi. They can also help the bronchial congestion of chest infections or asthma and combine well with Red Clover blossoms for spasmodic croup. Their diuretic effect enhances elimination through the kidneys and relieves fluid retention. Elderflowers relax the nerves and encourage a healing rest, particularly helpful for restless children. They can be taken as part of a spring cure, enhancing resistance and detoxifying blood and skin. Cold Elderflower tea can help reduce night sweats and menopausal flushes.

Fresh Elderflower pollen has been found helpful in the treatment of allergic conditions such as hay fever, rhinitis, and asthma. This can be collected from the flowers by placing the blossoms upside down on a sheet of glass overnight. The collected pollen can be stored in an airtight container and taken in small amounts daily.

Topically the flowers are anti-inflammatory and are used in skin creams and as an ointment for chilblains. The cold, strained infusion is useful as an eyewash for inflamed or sore eyes and can also combine well with Sage as a mouthwash and gargle for mouth ulcers, sore throats, and tonsillitis. As a skin lotion, Elderflowers cool sunburn, heal chilblains, and will both whiten and soften the skin.

Elderberries have similar properties to the flowers although they are less effective for bringing down fevers. The berries are antiviral and support the immune system, being rich in vitamins A and C. They make a delicious syrup and are taken to prevent and treat winter colds and to maintain a healthy heart and circulation. The juice is a useful remedy for long-standing rheumatism, neuralgia, and sciatica. The berries are laxative if large quantities are taken raw.

The fresh leaves, which should only be used externally, are soothing and wound healing. They can also relieve nervous headaches if warmed and laid on the temples. An infused oil of the leaves is helpful for piles (hemorrhoids) and can be used to make the once popular Green Elder Ointment, used for bruises, sprains, wounds, and piles. As an ointment the leaves are reported to have antitumor activity.

The bark has a reputation as a purgative but is generally considered too violent for internal use. It can be made into an ointment for rheumatism using the second year twigs, but this is rarely used in modern times.

## Additional Uses of Elder

Elder is harvested for commercial use and made into cordials, wine, and champagne. It has a range of additional culinary uses: the flower heads are fried in batter (Elderflower fritters); dried blossoms are used to make a flower vinegar; flowers and fruits are made into ketchup, jellies, and jams (especially good with Apples or Gooseberries); flowers are cooked with stewed fruit; young green shoots are pickled or boiled as a vegetable; juice is boiled with sugar to make Elderberry syrup, known as a "rob," and flavored with ginger and cloves. In France, pears are put to ripen on layers of Elder blossoms to impart a muscatel scent. When storing apples, Elder blossoms are placed among them to help them keep longer.

For cosmetic use the flowers are made into skin lotions or used as Elderflower water. Berries steeped in vinegar are also used as a black hair dye. In horticulture, the leaves are boiled and strained to make a natural insecticidal spray. For music, Elder twigs can be made into hollow flutes by removing the central white pith.

## PLANT DIETING WITH ELDER

*After choosing to diet Elder, it is time to harvest the plants and prepare your elixir. Below you will find recipes for two Elder elixirs that I made at Derrynagittah. I have described the instructions that I received from*

*Elder for making these two elixirs. When making your own elixir you will need to listen carefully to the plants and let them guide you. See chapter 4 for more complete information on harvesting plants and preparing the elixir.*

*In advance of your plant diet it is important to prepare yourself for several days with a period of physical and spiritual purification. At Derrynagittah we make specific cleansing and dietary recommendations for each diet. You will find the recommended preparations for the Elder diet below.*

## 🌿 MAKING THE ELDER ELIXIR

You will notice that while most components in the elixir recipes below are expressed as parts of the whole, certain ingredients (notably vibrational essences) are listed with a specific quantity. In these cases, the amount is NOT proportional to the total amount of elixir and represents a quantity simply added to the whole. This is an intuitive, guided choice and the amount can remain the same, regardless of total quantity; that is, the same number of drops of essence can be added, whether to 20 oz. of elixir or 2 gallons.

*Elixir I*
- I part Elderflower champagne
- I part Elderberry syrup

**Amount of elixir taken at diet:** Seven servings of 3 tablespoons and I teaspoon (50 ml) for each person

### Making the Elderflower Champagne

For the Elderflower champagne, flower heads were picked at the Summer Solstice and processed using a simple recipe:
- 4 handfuls of Elderflowers
- The juice of 2 lemons, plus grated zest
- 2 tablespoons of white wine vinegar
- 1.5 pounds sugar

Bring 40 fluid ounces of water to a boil, add sugar, and stir for a few minutes until syrupy. Remove from heat and put in a fermentation bucket. Top with cold water up to one gallon. Add remaining ingredients, stirring well. Cover and leave for two days, squeezing occasionally. Strain, and bottle in sterilized, screw-top bottles. Leave to mature for at least two months in a cool, dark place.

## Making the Elderberry Syrup

For the syrup, the Elderberries were harvested at the Autumn Equinox and processed by the following method:

De-stalk the Elderberries (a few handfuls will give a pint or so of juice). Take a large pan and add just enough water to cover the bottom of the pan. Place this over low heat and add the berries, a handful at a time, crushing them in the pan with the end of a rolling pin and being careful not to boil them. Keep doing this until all the berries are crushed. Let cool slightly and press out the juice through muslin. Return the juice to the clean pan adding 1 pound of honey per 20 oz. of liquid. Stir over gentle heat until dissolved. Allow to cool and pour into clean bottles.

For the Elder initiation outlined here I also used a Green Elder Oil for anointing the participants. This oil was made during the summer by boiling fresh Elder leaves in three times their volume of olive oil. The process was carried out at the time of a good friend's passing. I had just returned from visiting her, seriously ill, in England and although she was in a different country, I was informed by Elder that by making and using the oil I could support her transition. The oil provided a tangible psychic connection that I was able to utilize as part of my vigil. My friend passed with great beauty and I am forever grateful for the assistance of the Elder Mother. I was instructed to save the remaining oil for use at the forthcoming Elder initiation ceremony.

## *Elixir 2*

- ☙ 3 parts Elderflower champagne
- ☙ 2 parts Elderberry syrup
- ☙ 1 part maceration of fresh flowers in Delice de Sureau*
- ☙ 3 parts infusion of dried elderflowers
- ☙ 9 drops Elderflower essence

---

*Delice de Sureau is an artisanal Elderflower liqueur from France. Here the flowers had been infused in the liqueur for four months.

**Amount of elixir taken at diet:** Six servings of 3 tablespoons and 1 teaspoon (50 ml) for each person

For this elixir the champagne and the syrup were made through the same methods described above. I also picked a handful of fresh Elderflowers in July and added them to a bottle of Delice de Sureau, an Elderflower drink from Paris. The blossoms were left to macerate for four months, then strained out and discarded on the day of the final mixing when I incorporated a little of the fortified Delice de Sureau plus an infusion of dried Elderflowers and the Elderflower essence. This mixing was a very sacred ceremony where I felt the potent presence and deep healing of a circle of Grandmothers.

##  PREPARATION FOR THE ELDER PLANT DIET

### General Preparations
For three days prior to diet take NO refined sugar, added salt, meat or dairy products, strong spices, coffee, alcohol, or fermented foods. Avoid oils apart from olive oil. Do not engage in sexual activity.

### Food during the Elder Diet
For those not fasting we recommend apples and sunflower seeds.

### Suggested Drinks
We recommend Fennel or Ginger tea, and hot or cold water.

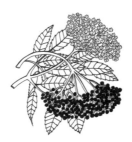

# DREAMING WITH ELDER

*Through the alchemy of sacred ceremony and by surrendering to the plant, participants in a plant diet enter into an altered state in which they form close relationships with the plant that they are dieting and receive gifts that*

may be physical, emotional, mental, and spiritual. Many participants gain a completely new perspective on life. The relationship with the plant is deeply transformative, facilitating access to higher consciousness, guidance, and healing. In this section people who have dieted with Elder tell the stories of their personal transformations.

## Gentleness and Sweetness

The Elder initiations have been notable for their gentleness. Maura described her time with Elder as "deep and profound, yet so gentle," while Camilla shared:

> It was a very gentle experience for me. I was just feeling and calling to the Elder to unveil only a little bit, for me not to try too hard, just to hold a space to uncover a little. This felt very appropriate because of the Elder's gentle and feminine nature. This is the way the tree is with its blossoms, which are more like a flower plant. The leaves are arranged in a delicate way; the blossom is very feminine, like old lace; and the berries have a delicate way of presenting themselves.

For Brenda, Elder evoked the qualities of a kindly witch. She recalled, "I received powerful healing and I was aware of so much kindness and support, sweetness and wisdom. It really showed me the sweetness of the old wizened crone or witch and how being a witch can be such an amazingly beautiful healing thing." Most participants referred to the crone or wise old woman aspect of the Elder, however Erica chose to spend time with a young plant and her experience "was not of an old woman but of a very gracious, very beautiful, and elegant plant, more of a younger woman, simple and humble."

## Physical Healing

The Elder diets facilitated healing of many physical complaints. Marie related how she had been "plagued with sinusitis and headaches for weeks prior to the initiation." She went on to say that she "asked the Elder for healing and halfway through the weekend I realized my headache was gone and it didn't come back." Jane experienced relief from a long-standing back problem. She gave this account:

*Coming here I expected to connect with Elder on a spiritual level but what I did not expect is that my spine has been affected. My back has been stiff and at times very sore for the past year. Each time I drank the elixir I felt a freeing up in my spine. Then after doing the GreenBreath with Elder I nearly jumped up, the back stiffness and pain were gone. It was the first time I felt like this in a year. It was very sore again through the night but I asked Elder to help and it eased. To me the physical effect of Elder on the spine has to do with its freeing quality. It felt like it was about freeing, releasing.*

Several months later, Jane commented, "the Elder diet has had a lasting effect physically: one of the ways in which it had an effect was on my back. I remember that I was having problems with my lower back for at least a year and overall it has gotten much better since the Elder initiation. I feel very grateful to Elder."

## *Opening Gateways to the Otherworld: Coming Home*

Images of gateways, veils, doors, and windows were common with Elder. Maura related, "All weekend I have been seeing windows—in journeys, in dreams, and noticing the windows of the buildings here. I cannot express it in words, but there is something big going on with windows for me. It feels like I'm being shown a completely new place that I've never seen before." Brenda described "the beauty of going into the world of the Elder, going behind the veil and being shown what we can bring through from there. Also I was seeing a lot of plant life looking so radiant and colors that I don't even know, a world that is shiny and pristine and full of crystals combined with plants."

Erica experienced a coming together of two parts of herself:

*The weekend felt like a homecoming and meeting with the Elder was like coming home, reconnecting with somebody I have known for a long time.*

*I realize there is a synthesis happening, a coming together of two parts,*
*combining the intuitive and the logical aspects of myself. It doesn't have to*
*be one or the other, they both come together.*

Erica also felt a link between Elder and the Sheela na gigs of Ireland,[*]
saying, "The Elder took me to a cavern underground and along a path that
came to a Sheela na gig or *Síle na gCíoch*. I saw the connection between
Elder and the Sheela na gig. Later in the GreenBreath, she came to me
again and I realized I was lying with my legs wide apart and my hands on
my breasts."

## Sexual Energy

Several participants mentioned sexual encounters with Elder, frequently
giving accounts of the clearing of blocked sexual energy and the reclaiming of sexual power. Dalton described the diet as a "sexual weekend"
and recalled how he had met Elder in the form of a "typical crone" or
old woman. She invited him to embrace her, and when he did so, he was
astounded to find that she had transformed into a young and beautiful
maiden. For Emma, Elder came to her as a male lover, while Michele
described her encounter with Elder as "carnal" and recounted how she was
"caressed and stroked in an intimate dance with Elder."

## Letting Go and Creating a New Reality

The freeing and releasing qualities that Jane described earlier were echoed
by Bridget, who shared that for her the Elder was a powerful ally helping her to let go of something she found particularly difficult. During the
weekend of her initiation we held a Samhain fire where we each made and
burnt an effigy from sticks and grasses representing all that we intended to
release from the old year. Bridget recounted:

---

[*]Sheela na Gigs are carvings of naked women displaying an exaggerated vulva. They are
found on churches, castles, and other buildings, most notably in Ireland, but also in Britain and some other countries as well. In Ireland they are often interpreted as *Síle na*
*gCíoch* (Sheila of the Breasts) and seen to represent the crone aspect of the Celtic Goddess Trinity of maiden, mother, and crone.

*The burning of the effigies was very powerful and I felt a huge freedom from the burning of mine. It seemed like an authentic letting go of attachments and yet the next day I was still asking the Elder for release of the blockage in my throat. The Elder said, "You have to believe that it is possible." I realized that I believed I was stuck with this block and it was not possible for me to be free of it. Even if I released it, I kept calling it back. The Elder told me to make another effigy. I was instructed to put my old belief into a clay figure, to bury it, and then the earth would compost it. So I sat with some clay, doing my best to stay as present as possible with my feelings and beliefs and to let them pour out of my hands into the clay figure. I also did a painting of my throat with all the pain, knives, blood, blackness, and fighting . . . I added essences for extra help and then I wrapped everything up together, ready for burying. I dug a hole at the feet of the Elder behind the herb garden and buried the figure and the picture, together with a sprig of Rue for extra cleansing. Having been at the last Blackthorn initiation, dieting now with the Elder felt like a perfect progression. For me the Blackthorn pierced a lot of karmic issues and some of it I held on to. The time in between has been useful for being with that, for trusting that whatever story I tell myself is somehow serving my evolution and growth process; for accepting it fully without trying to fix, control, deny, or judge; for trusting the darkness. Now the Elder has come along with death and letting go, releasing and healing. Both plants are amazing ancient beings. I perceive them both as Grandmothers.*

The significance of our beliefs and expectations was a common theme. Erica echoed the sentiment: "I addressed a number of things and I was expecting resistance or difficulty. The question was, 'could I allow it to be that easy?'" Jane revealed, "This whole experience with the Elder has made me aware of my limitations. I feel my head is limiting me. I tend to over-think things. This is one of my limitations. Letting go is important." For Joan, a dream illustrated how easy it can be to change our reality:

*I dreamed that I had finished work and I was coming down the corridor when I realized I needed to shut down a computer. When I looked at the screen it was in a foreign language and I couldn't understand it. A friend's husband suggested I look up the manual. Shortly after that I found the exit key and each screen, as I shut it down, was a different situation in my life. All I had to do was exit it to close it down. I realized that it is that simple to shut down my dramas—just hit the exit button.*

## Connecting with Ancestors

As outlined above, at one of the diets described here I used Green Elder Oil to anoint the third eye of the initiates. This helped to draw their consciousness to this energy center and facilitated their inner seeing along with the presence of Elder. Even without using an oil, our inner vision is particularly open around Samhain and there is an easy connection with the ancestors. Dieting with Elder at this time of year amplifies this effect and is a potent way to meet with the ancestors and to facilitate ancestral healing.

Jane recalled, "I did feel the presence of the ancestors. I felt very in touch with my grandparents. A different thing was that I could see and hear them and it was beautiful." Camilla explained how she met with her deceased grandparents and was looking at the gifts they had passed on to her:

*Last night I met my four grandparents, who are all dead, trying to fathom their gifts to me. One I never met. They came and spoke individually. There were certain aspects of themselves that I viewed a little differently. They had all bestowed gifts and I was looking at anything that needed to be cleared and might be impacting relationships in my own life. Just at the very end a Celtic shaman appeared from my grandfather's lineage from Ulster and revealed that there is a shamanic tradition in the family. I slept well and felt that the whole process was gentle. I felt the connection with the Elder and with the snake shedding its skins.*

Patricia also connected with an ancestor. She met her deceased father and asked if he needed healing for any reason. "He told me that he always lacked confidence in his life and I realized that self-confidence is one of the core issues that my soul has come to learn in this lifetime. The Elder can help me heal this for myself as well as for the generations behind me and those still to come."

Our ancestors include our blood family through time as well as those with whom we have a spiritual connection. Bridget shared that during the weekend she experienced the strong presence of a circle of spiritual Grandmothers. She was not sure of their identity but she said, "they are definitely connected with the Elder and it seems to me that we are all being asked to remember something from the Grandmothers and to bring it forth into our lives."

Brenda's dreaming with Elder brought her in touch with her maternal grandmother:

*I am in a house in a time in the past and there's an open trap door leading to a secret basement. I go down the stairs and into this basement where there's a red liquid waiting to be drunk—I know it's the Elder. The liquid is in a clear glass bottle on a wooden table and there's a wooden chair. I have a sense of Biddy Early being here and then I notice that my grandmother is here in a rocking chair.\* In the dream I know her well even though she died before I was born. She tells me I must value myself and what I do. She says that she didn't value herself and it gave her cancer. She is knitting a patchwork and she gives me a knitted heart. Then I drink the liquid and my chest starts moving and I feel it fluttering. I go to a barred window. A pure white bird emerges from my heart and out of my chest. It's a mixture of a dove and an eagle. I open the window and free the bird into the world—sad to see it go but happy to see it free. It flies toward the sun, which is big and hot, and as the bird gets closer it begins to melt, becoming stickier and stickier as it gets nearer to the sun. I feel distraught watching it melt. The next thing I know, I am in a meadow of daisies. I am the same size as them and it is absolutely beautiful. Golden drops are falling out of the sky instead of raindrops and I know it is the golden drops from the bird after being transformed. She says, "I never left. I am always here. I never*

*Biddy Early (1798–1874) was a renowned Irish healer and wise woman from County Clare.

*left you." I feel wonderful, dancing with joy among the enormous daisies
and receiving the Light from the drops of gold.*

Brenda later commented:

*There's a lot in this dream—the presence of my grandmother and her
message about valuing myself and how not doing so is a family pattern.
The bird symbolized purity and strength for me. I feel it's about letting go
and allowing myself to transform. The dream is also showing me how much
help I have and how I am never alone—that separation is just an illusion.
There's a lot for me to be with.*

## Children and Death: Transforming Grief

Given that Elder is such a helpful medicine for children, it is probably
not surprising how often babies and children were mentioned at the Elder
diets. Sometimes this related to the loss of a child, reflecting how Elder
assists with death and letting go as well as connecting us with our ancestors. Furthermore, during one of our Elder initiations, Naira, a member
of our original group who had previously attended numerous plant diets,
gave birth in a hospital to a baby boy. To date, this is the only time that
one of our group has given birth during a plant initiation and there was a
beautiful synchronicity in the way that this took place while the rest of us
were holding for her in our circle with the Elder Mother.

For Emer, a significant message from Elder was that "I have to go
home and maintain the peace, to be the peace. It's something important
I have to give to the four boys [her sons]. I have to rear them in the right
way." Barbara shared:

*The main thing that came up was the importance of children, and dead
children came up too. I have five children and I had an abortion and a
miscarriage that I never acknowledged. I feel it is past-life stuff too. I have
heard about children who died at the breast during the Famine. I feel that
is part of who I am. I found the GreenBreath powerful. Children came up
again. There was a lot of grief and also incredible gratitude—gratitude to*

*my parents, whom I did not have a great relationship with on and off, and gratitude for the five children I have. I am just hoping they will be all right. I do not mind as long as they are okay. I am glad for this weekend. I feel different now.*

Jane recounted:

*Something regarding children came up during a journey with the Elder. I do not have children. I had a miscarriage and we did in vitro fertilization a year ago and it did not work. I did not think it was still such an issue. But it was a major issue for a long time. I felt major healing here two months ago. I felt much ease from what I experienced here and I still do. I felt big joy from thinking I can let go of not having a child—it is not my path, there are things I can do to contribute to this world. For years, wanting a child has put a limit to anything I wanted to do. There are other ways I can contribute to the Earth, especially around plants. On one of my journeys I felt my tummy open and I felt this presence of a child. I felt I was connecting to the miscarriage and the IVF. The image was very big and then dissolved into the energy of a small circle. I did ask the faeries for some help and for healing. Airmid came and put her hands on my belly.\* I think it was her. I kept asking for more karmic release. I kept very positive.*

Mary Teresa, whose elder son was killed in a traffic accident, explained that her intent for the weekend was to bring healing to her other son, "to relieve him of the burden of grief he has been carrying for the last few years. To transform the sadness and bring him healing; to free him." She describes her experience with Elder:

*I felt it begin when I was bringing the Elder into my light wheels. When I felt the Elder in my first light wheel, I instantly felt deeply connected to my son and as I felt the Elder in each light wheel I could feel the connection to him getting stronger and stronger.*

---

\*The goddess Airmid is a Tuatha de Danaan deity credited with knowing the secrets of herbalism.

*I am in a dream. One of my ancestors comes. He shows me my son lying on the ground. There are old women gathered round him, faces wizened with age. At first I worry that there is something wrong with him, but I trust my ancestor and he tells me all is right. One woman seems to take over and starts painting symbols on his body. When she starts this I find myself in his body reliving many memories from the past. Memories of when his brother died, those days after the funeral. One memory sticks out. I am him, carrying his brother's coffin. My right ear is next to the coffin. I am listening. I can feel his body through the coffin as we carry it to the grave. I am confused. How can he be dead? What does it mean? We cannot put him in the ground. I feel the grief, the loss. Many more memories come, all difficult to bear. I am back in the other scene. The old woman is washing his body now. He looks at peace. She then rubs oil onto his body. When she is finished she draws the outline of a body beside him in the dirt. It is a woman and she comes to life. Her hair is long and flowing, streaked of all different colors: black, white, grey, red, blonde, and brown. She begins to dance around his body for some time as if in ceremony. The scene changes. I see him sitting on the ground in front of his brother. Both of their faces are painted like warriors. I can see their energies touch and something opens between them. Images begin to emerge. Images of them running as boys together, running as men together, running together in different lifetimes. He is back lying on the ground again. The woman is still dancing around him. She takes his hand and they begin to dance. Sometimes the dance is wild but they move perfectly together. Sometimes her face changes and I see the face of his best friend—I clearly see her beautiful face. They dance and dance for what seems like a long time. The image changes. My younger son is sitting on a throne, he is dressed in gold with a headband of gold. There is a woman sitting next to him, also dressed in gold and there is a child on his knee.*

Inspired by Elder, Mary Teresa shared the following poem:

> *Two brothers together,*
> *We ran through life.*

*Supporting each other*
*Through fun and through strife.*

*Starting from childhood,*
*Just two little boys.*
*We stuck together*
*As we played with our toys.*

*Acting out the characters*
*We would love to be,*
*Where would life bring us?*
*What was the key?*

*I played guitar;*
*You played the drums.*
*We would start with our music*
*And see what comes.*

*You were my hero,*
*I looked up to you.*
*I watched you closely,*
*In all you would do.*

*We could not wait to*
*Learn to drive,*
*Then we would really*
*Be alive.*

*You started first,*
*Being older then me.*
*So you drove me around,*
*We had much to see.*

*You were always*
*The careful one,*
*Though you still knew*
*How to have fun.*

*I waited for you*
*On that last night,*
*But all was still*
*And all too quiet.*

*Playing your music*
*As you drove along,*
*The last thing you heard*
*Was your favorite song.*

*Gone forever*
*My brother my friend,*
*We never thought*
*This is how it would end.*

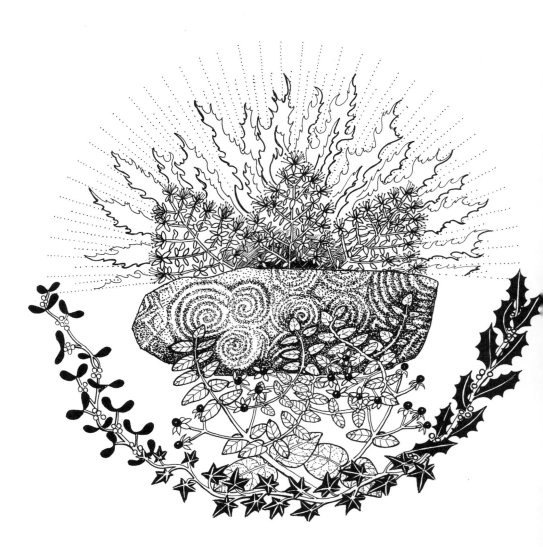

*At the Winter Solstice—the shortest day of the year—we
celebrate the return of the light.*

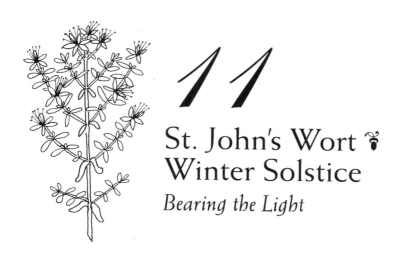

# 11
# St. John's Wort 🐝
# Winter Solstice
## *Bearing the Light*

*S*ince ancient times, St. John's Wort has been associated with the Light. Its bright yellow flowers symbolize the sun and it has the power to cast out negativity and dispel darkness (see color plate 9). A long-recognized "herbe of protection," in medieval England St. John's Wort was revered as a magical talisman capable of protecting from evil influences, healing disease, and bringing good luck. Ruled by the sun and corresponding to the astrological sign of Leo, this herb was traditionally linked with Sun Gods, Midsummer's Day, and the element of Fire. With the coming of Christianity, the plant was rededicated to St. John the Baptist, and Midsummer's Day became St. John's Day, credited as being the date of John's birth. Christians refer to St. John as the precursor of Jesus, the forerunner who prepares the way and announces Jesus's coming. It is no coincidence that St. John should be linked to this herb. St. John's Wort, with its bright saffron-colored flowers, is the epitome of a Light carrier and the prophet of a coming Golden Age. This plant, which recent research shows is a protector against the modern "demons" of depression and viral illness, is helping to lead humanity into the Light.

Previously, I associated St. John's Wort with the Summer rather than the Winter Solstice, yet recent events have given me a new perspective that I will explain below. These events made the resolute St. John's Wort my clear choice of plant to feature for the Winter Solstice in this book. In 2012, during the months approaching the Winter Solstice, I began to have dreams about St. John's Wort in which the plant was carrying a new form of solar energy and was acting as a bridge between Heaven and Earth. In these dreams, St. John's Wort (particularly the Tutsan species,) revealed itself as a feisty pioneer, determined to bring new Light to the Earth while working in partnership with certain other plants.

I was taken inside the St. John's Wort cells and into the world of photosynthesis, which is the amazing process by which plants convert light energy (mainly from the sun) into chemical energy, stored as carbohydrates. I was shown how the green pigment chlorophyll receives light and uses it for energy transformation. In this case the chlorophyll in the plant cells was co-creating with the Emerald Ray and I received the powerful message that plants (in this instance led by St. John's Wort) can help humans to hold more Light and can activate our hearts. The Emerald Ray is one of several spiritual rays, each associated with a different color and carrying specific gifts on our planet. These rays can be accorded various meanings. For me, the Emerald Ray has an intimate connection with the heart (as well as with Ireland). It carries harmony, joy, and knowledge and is associated with the awakening and evolution of the heart. So, to reiterate, *plants can activate our hearts and they can help us to hold more Light.* What's more, they are actively pursuing this now. This is an astonishing gift. I do believe that our hearts hold the answer to humanity's awakening, and considering that the plant world gives us life, and has helped forge our evolutionary path, it makes perfect sense to me that plants are involved in helping us to transform our hearts. Amazing as it may seem—despite human actions—the plant world continues to offer us love and generosity. Plants are doing their very best to help us move forward. Thus it became clear that St. John's Wort had a significant role to play during the 2012 Winter Solstice, which was a major planetary gateway. I subsequently included the plant when making my Solstice flower essence and during the days around the Solstice I observed St. John's Wort closely.

My experience at the time was of the Tutsan species receiving and anchoring a new form of Light from our sun and passing this on to the other local St. John's Wort species. These plants then spread this new form of Light (or perhaps the ability to collect the Light) to other plants, animals, and receptive humans, seeming to pass it on by a form of resonance called entrainment, a phenomenon in which frequencies adjust to and align themselves with the frequency of a dominant stimulus. In the months following the Solstice, I was surprised to discover previously unseen Tutsan plants in key areas of the land here, while it also became increasingly widespread throughout the county. I am well aware that all has not yet been revealed on this matter, but my understanding at the time of writing is that the new Light on our planet can activate previously dormant DNA in all of us. This process is part of the evolution of our consciousness. St. John's Wort is playing a key role in the evolution of planet Earth. It has been carrying a new form of Light since the Winter Solstice of 2012, when it came forward as a Light bearer, offering to carry the new Light to other beings.

Successive dreams and meditations have indicated that the mitochondria of the cells (both plant and human) are particularly significant in the process of holding and spreading this new Light. Our mitochondrial "power packs" produce the energy in our bodies. They are also involved in producing light. We emit light in the form of biophotons, and most of these biophotons emerge from the DNA of our mitochondria. German scientist Fritz Popp* believes that these biophotons are an expression of our qi, an intelligent energy force. In addition to producing energy, the mitochondria are instrumental in facilitating programmed cell death, which means they not only allow our bodies to form in the womb but they are also implicated in diseases like cancer, where a healthy self-destruct mechanism fails to occur. Our mitochondria carry maternal

---

*F. A. Popp, "Properties of Biophotons and Their Theoretical Implications," *Indian Journal of Experimental Biology* 41 (5) (2003): 440–45.

DNA, anchoring the sacred feminine energy that is held by Shekinah (among others), which we work with here in the labyrinth. It is clear that mitochondria play a significant role in our evolution, and I believe a lot more will be learned and revealed about them in the near future.*

Returning to the subject of the new Light and our newly accessible DNA, these offer the potential to help us open and activate our hearts as a source of Divine Light. Through this process, all our cells can begin to emit more Light, giving an opportunity for our entire bodies to transform into Light. Working with the Emerald Ray, plants may help the heart to learn and remember how to both hold Light and to be an instrument of energy transformation. Perhaps, on the path to enlightenment, the human heart is learning how to photosynthesize!

## WINTER SOLSTICE
### *Rebirth of the Light*

The Winter Solstice is the shortest day and the longest night of the year in the Northern Hemisphere. Falling between December 20 and December 23, this is the festival of rebirth when we celebrate the rebirth of the sun and the return of the light after being in darkness. Otherwise known as Yule (*Jul*), which means "wheel" in Norwegian, this is when the Wheel of the Year stops and starts again. From now on the days will lengthen, bringing light and hope.

In past times (and still in places today), a Yule log was burned to help the sun shine more brightly. This log was received as a gift or gathered from the land (never bought) and decorated with greenery. It was burned at the Solstice and the ashes were kept for good fortune or sprinkled over the land to ensure fertility. A portion of the ashes were often kept for next year's Solstice fire to promote the harmonious turning of the wheel. In England, crops and trees were *wassailed* with toasts of spiced cider, blessing them with song or with the word *wassail,* which means "be whole" in Old English.

---

*Read *Power, Sex, Suicide: Mitochondria and the Meaning of Life* by Nick Lane for more information on these magnificent organelles (see bibliography).

Other Winter Solstice traditions are often still practiced in modern times. Evergreen plants, symbolizing everlasting life, are brought into the house as decoration, providing shelter for the nature spirits over the coldest months of winter. Mistletoe represents fertility and the seed of the Divine, being particularly held sacred if found growing on Oak trees. Holly opens the heart and honors the underworld goddess, while Ivy helps us follow our path to enlightenment. We can make a wreath of evergreens to represent the turning of the wheel.

The Winter Solstice is a time to celebrate with friends and family, expressing your generosity and gratitude. Light candles to welcome the new light. Let go of the old, gather your intent, and make resolutions for the future. Winter Solstice is a time of pause when Nature holds her breath for a moment before starting a new cycle. Take time to be still; take a break from everyday activities and simply be. There is a magical alchemy in greeting the Winter Solstice sunrise, honoring the returning light as was done by our ancestors at Newgrange in County Meath five thousand years ago. At this ancient cairn, a shaft of light illuminates the inner chamber at Winter Solstice, and today in Ireland this event is televised across the country.

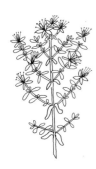

## ST. JOHN'S WORT—THE LIGHT BEARER
*Hypericum perforatum: Perforate St. John's Wort*

**Plant family:** Clusiaceae or Hypericaceae (St. John's Wort Family).

**Other common names:** Balm of Warriors; Penny John; Touch-and-Heal; Save; Herba John; Goat Weed; Tipton Weed; Klamath Weed; Amber; Bible Flower; Holy Herb.

**Description:** A hardy perennial growing to a height of one to three feet, it is erect and hairless with pairs of long-oval leaves that are ¼ to 1¼ inches long. The leaves are covered in translucent dots that look very much like tiny holes but are in fact oil glands. A good way to identify the correct species is to hold a leaf up to the sun and look for these "perforations."

The petals and sepals are also dotted with black glands, and the petals rubbed between the fingers will produce a red stain. Plants tolerate most soils and grow in both full sun and light shade, often self-seeding. They can be grown from seed sown in spring or propagated from runners in the autumn.

**Habitat:** Plants are found in open woodland, rough pasture, grassy banks, and waste ground.

**Distribution:** They are native to Europe, West Asia, and North Africa. While non-native to North America, they are widespread and considered naturalized throughout most of the United States.

**Species:** There are almost four hundred species of *Hypericum,* providing medicinal plants as well as garden plants such as Rose of Sharon (*Hypericum calycinum*). Apart from Tutsan (*Hypericum androsaemum*), most do not have as strong healing virtues as *Hypericum perforatum.* Tutsan, named from the French *Toute Saine,* or "Heal-all" (to be differentiated from *Prunella vulgaris,* which is commonly referred to as Heal-all or Self-heal), is an ancient healing plant reported to have similar medicinal properties to Perforate St. John's Wort. Tutsan is perennial and shrubby with reddish stems, five-petaled yellow flowers, and glossy berries, which turn from whitish green to red and finally to black. The flowers and seed heads are faintly aromatic when crushed. Native to open woods and hillsides in Eurasia, it has become an invasive weed in parts of North and South America, Australasia, and South Africa. This has not occurred to the same extent in Europe and can be viewed as a sign of the dangers of human interference with the balance of ecology. Perforate St John's Wort is also considered invasive in some areas. In 1946 in northern California, leaf beetles were introduced to control the spread of Perforate St. John's Wort. These insects have a voracious appetite for the plant and by 1957 the stands of *Hypericum* were reduced to 1 percent of their original number. Another perspective on invasive plants is given by Timothy Lee Scott in his book *Invasive Plant Medicine: The Ecological Benefits and Healing Abilities of Invasives,* where he shares a message received through a plant dream. His dream intimates that inva-

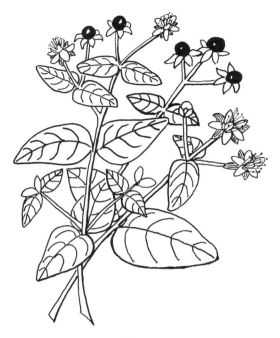

*Tutsan*

sive plants are serving the evolution of planet Earth by helping to "stabilize habitats and create integrity within the landscape." He suggests that such plants are "transform[ing] industrial runoff, pharmaceutical pollution, and other toxic pollutants."*

**Parts used:** Herb and flowering tops (fresh or dried), preferably gathered on a sunny day during flowering. For medicinal use, Tutsan and Perforate St. John's Wort may be used interchangeably.

## St. John's Wort as a Spirit Medicine

As a spirit medicine, St. John's Wort is a major Light bringer. It increases a person's sensitivity to spiritual Light, helping the person to know and radiate the Light of his or her own soul. St. John's Wort brings a remarkable

---

*Timothy Lee Scott, *Invasive Plant Medicine: The Ecological Benefits and Healing Abilities of Invasives* (Rochester, Vt.: Healing Arts Press, 2010), 89.

amount of Light into our bodies and helps us to absorb Light by enhancing our receptivity to it. It has the effect of awakening and activating the Light within and it facilitates profound healing and personal development by helping us to remember who we are as spiritual beings. Along with this comes the remembrance of the huge amount of spiritual help available, including the recollection of spirit guides and allies. St. John's Wort activates our DNA, transforms us on a cellular level, and encourages self-love. It helps bring our bodies, cells, and DNA into a healthy resonance. It sends Light into the darkness, transforming fear and dark thoughts while giving rise to feelings of safety, strength, confidence, and illumination. St. John's Wort exerts a spiritual influence on the third eye and can thereby awaken visionary experiences and promote awareness of multi-dimensionality.

The plant provides a fine example of the intimate connection between physical and spiritual. From molecular biology and the study of biophotons, we know that our body cells communicate via light in an electromagnetic field. Our tissues and organs are highly organized structures in which the cells are constantly communicating via light and this communication is one of the bridges to consciousness. It is a connecting link between our physical and spiritual selves. Light is crucial to healing and to life itself. We know that all plants carry Light, yet St. John's Wort is a supreme case in point. The fact that this plant is bringing *so* much Light to humans is of massive significance to our healing and to the evolution of human consciousness. St. John's Wort is literally leading us toward en*light*enment. St. John's Wort is greatly participating in the current planetary shift in consciousness and it is no surprise that awareness of this plant has become so heightened around the world at this point in history.

At the Summer Solstice St. John's Wort brings cleansing and protection and celebrates the sun's power. It is also highly appropriate at the Winter Solstice to welcome and honor the return of the Light. All year round it is used to connect with the Sun and to commune with the spirits of Fire.

## St. John's Wort as a Flower Essence

**Key words to describe this essence:**
Protection and light.

The essence of St. John's Wort brings divine protection, spiritual guidance, and feelings of safety. It helps us to know the Light within, to hold and anchor that Light, and to radiate it out to others. St. John's Wort is especially valuable for sensitive people who are spiritually open. It is beneficial for those who fear psychic attack and also when taken before sleep to prevent nightmares. It makes a good addition to essence sprays for protection.

## St. John's Wort in Folklore and History

St. John's Wort has been used as a medicine since antiquity. Considered a powerful healer and protector by the ancient Greeks, the plant was prescribed by Hippocrates, Dioscorides, and Pliny for a wide range of conditions from burns to bladder conditions, pleurisy to insanity. In the Middle Ages, St. John's Wort was highly prized in the treatment of septic wounds and burns. It was also used to expel bile and urine, to stimulate menstruation, and to cure sciatica and gout. Nicholas Culpeper reported that St. John's Wort "opens obstructions, dissolves swellings, and closes up the lips of wounds." Popular folk uses included internal treatments for kidney stones, ulcerations of the kidneys, fevers, jaundice, gout, rheumatism, and chronic catarrh of the lung, bowels, or urinary passages. A warm lotion was made for injuries to the spinal cord, damaged nerves, bed sores, and lock jaw as well. It was widely recommended for insanity and hypochondria. In these cases, the fresh plant was bound to the forehead to banish dark thoughts. It was said to bring Light to a distressed heart and "rainbow visions" to the mind, the latter hinting at its visionary qualities. The crusaders used St. John's Wort to heal their wounds and from this it got its folk name, Save, as an all-healing herb for sword wounds.

The name *Hypericum* is derived from the Greek *hyperikon* meaning "over an apparition" due to its renowned ability to protect against negative influences. A sprig of the plant was placed above the icon or picture of a person or thing to be charmed, usually against evil spirits. In fact, it was said that St. John's Wort was so detested by evil spirits that they would fly off at a whiff of its odor. Formerly, the plant was called *Fuga Doemoniorum* (Scare Devil), Devil's Scourge, Grace of God, Lord God's Wonder Plant, and other similar names. Throughout Europe, the plant was used for protection against evil. It was eaten, worn as an amulet, placed under the pillow at night, and planted in the four corners of a house or field. In Germany, an extract of consecrated Perforate St. John's Wort was poured into a baby's first bath. It was also known as Witch's Herb and reputed to be used by witches to help them hear spirits. Like many magical plants, it was sometimes used for countermagic. During the witch hunts, a piece of St. John's Wort was placed into the mouths of people accused of witchcraft in the belief that it would make them confess. Similarly, at the early witch trials a potion was made from St. John's Wort and Thistle seed and given to suspected witches to break the power of the Devil and force the person (who had also been tortured) to speak the truth.

St. John's Wort flowers around the Summer Solstice and all over Europe it was traditionally burned in the Midsummer fires to cast off trouble and misfortune. The smoke was wafted over houses and fields and the plant was hung in doorways, windows, and under eaves for purification and protection from illness, lightning, and all kinds of negativity. In medieval times the red oil and yellow flowers were seen as symbols of blood and solar fire, while ancient Druids considered the plant a perfect combination of fire and water. In Germanic mythology the red juice is seen as the blood of Balder, the Germanic God of Nature, Summer, and Light, and the son of Odin and Freya. Christianity replaced Balder with St. John the Baptist and the juice then became known as St. John's Blood, which for many years was considered a magic potion. In Holland, the common names were *Sint-Jans-bloed* (St John's Blood) and *Johannesbloed* (John's Blood). St. John's feast day falls on June 24 during the period of the old Midsummer feast. Among the Christian saints St. John represents Light. Throughout Europe, the yellow blooms of St. John's Wort were seen as a reminder of the beneficent sun and the apparent holes in the leaves signified John's wounds. Harvested on St. John's Day, the flowers were soaked in olive oil to produce an anointing oil called the Blood of Christ, also known as Heart of Jesus Oil.

In England, to prevent children's nightmares and aid restful sleep, a sprig of St. John's Wort was placed with dried Thyme inside a mattress. Similarly, to sleep on a pillow of St. John's Wort and Sage was thought to give prophetic dreams, while rubbing dried leaves on wrists or temples was known to relieve stress. For protection, a sprig of St. John's Wort was carried when traveling alone at night. The plant was also a fertility remedy and the red juice was used in love potions since the time of the ancient Greeks. In medieval England it was said that if a childless woman walked naked to pick St. John's Wort, she could expect to conceive within the year. In the 1930s in Croatia, an infertile woman would drink an extract of Perforate St. John's Wort that had first been consecrated by a priest. And in Friuli, Italy, the plant is still regarded as an aphrodisiac today.

The plant was frequently used for divination, for every situation from longevity to romance. To predict their chances for marital bliss, young girls would pluck a sprig of St. John's Wort. If the flowers were fresh in the morning, their chances were good; if wilted, a dismal outcome was predicted. This poem is translated from the German, where this custom was also practiced:

> The young maid stole through the cottage door,
> And blushed as she sought the plant of power.
> 'Thou silver glow-worm, oh! lend me thy light,
> I must gather the mystic St. John's Wort to-night;
> The wonderful herb whose leaf will decide
> If the coming year shall see me a bride.

In the Victorian language of flowers, St. John's Wort says, "The shining of your spirit has captured my heart."

## St. John's Wort in Contemporary Herbal Medicine

St. John's Wort is a highly precious herbal medicine, used primarily in my practice as a strengthening tonic for the nervous system and as an antiviral remedy. It lifts the spirits, eases anxiety, and calms the nerves, making it helpful for stress, excitability, sleep problems, and obsessive compulsive disorder. As an antidepressant it affects neurotransmitters in the brain and can be of lasting benefit when taken for at least two months.

This plant has been called the Arnica of the nervous system, reflecting its powerful healing influence on our nerves when affected by shock and trauma.* It is particularly helpful for injuries to flesh with a rich nerve supply, such as fingertips and the soles of the feet. St. John's Wort relieves postoperative pain, reduces the pain of dental extraction, and is useful for concussion. Its affinity with the nervous system combined with its pain-relieving and anti-inflammatory actions make it helpful for neuralgia and rheumatic pain including sciatica. St. John's Wort treats muscle pain and fibromyalgia as well as earache, toothache, and nervous headache. It is a useful herb for women; beneficial for painful, heavy periods, for PMS, and for anxiety and mood changes at menopause. It treats restless leg syndrome and in terminal disease it can relieve cramps while supporting the nervous system. The plant's antiviral activity makes it a highly valuable remedy in the treatment of viruses and it is one of the best herbs for treating shingles and other herpes infections, strengthening the nerves and speeding tissue repair.

St. John's Wort is a gentle decongestant for the liver and gallbladder and can be used in the treatment of gallstones. It assists in the detoxification of the body when toxicity is caused by pharmaceutical drugs. It strengthens the digestion, normalizing stomach acid and improving the absorption of nutrients. Astringent and antibacterial, it can relieve gastroenteritis and diarrhea. A diuretic and tonic for the urinary system, St. John's Wort reduces mild fluid retention and is used to treat bedwetting in children, nervous bladder, and stress incontinence. It is also a gentle expectorant, clearing mucus from the respiratory system and relieving irritable coughs. Because it contains melatonin, it helps to prevent and treat jet lag and may have an effect on the pineal gland.† St. John's Wort

---

*Arnica is a powerful herb used externally for shock and injury. It is used internally as a homeopathic medicine.

†Melatonin is a hormone produced by the pineal gland that promotes healthy sleep patterns by entraining the body with Nature's circadian rhythms.

makes an excellent combination with Oats for depression, anxiety, nerve damage, or shingles. It combines well with Echinacea, Garlic, and Elderberry for viral illness and with Mugwort or Milk Thistle for liver support.

In Europe in the 1990s, St. John's Wort shot to fame as an herbal antidepressant. This was due to the publication of scientific studies that showed extracts of the plant to be at least as effective as certain pharmaceutical antidepressants (known as SSRIs or Selective Serotonin Reuptake Inhibitors) yet without the unwanted side effects of these drugs. St. John's Wort rapidly became a popular over-the-counter herbal remedy and outsold Prozac by a factor of seven to one.* Today St. John's Wort is one of the world's most widely used herbal supplements, representing a massive global industry. A drawback of these over-the-counter proprietary herbal medicines is that they are frequently standardized on a marker compound (often considered the main "active ingredient") and are therefore different from the whole plant as it occurs in nature with its complex mix of constituents. This man-made change may cause the medicine to be associated with idiosyncratic effects, which are less likely to occur with a whole-plant preparation such as a simple infusion or tincture.

St. John's Wort is significant in helping us to absorb light. It is beneficial for those with S.A.D. (Seasonal Affective Disorder) where people are adversely affected by a lack of sunlight in the winter months. It is interesting to note that the plant has been known to produce an oversensitivity to sunlight in cattle and sheep when they have consumed large quantities and then spent long periods in the sun. This is known as photosensitivity and people taking the herb are sometimes advised to avoid sunbathing in case they develop skin irritation. There have been no verifiable human cases recorded although some adverse effects have been reported from over-the-counter preparations.

A very real caution exists with St. John's Wort if you are taking pharmaceutical drugs. The plant efficiently helps the body to remove toxins.

---

*The antidepressant Prozac is a widely prescribed proprietary form of Citalopram (Celexa), an SSRI drug.

This includes promoting the removal of certain pharmaceutical medications and potentially reducing their effectiveness. For safety, do not take St. John's Wort with any pharmaceutical medication without first getting advice from an herbal practitioner.

Externally St. John's Wort is used as an infused oil, ointment, or lotion, which can be made from either an infusion or a tincture. The oil is made by filling a clear glass jar with chopped, fresh flowering tops and covering them with cold-pressed oil, preferably olive or sunflower. Leave this in a closed jar in bright sunlight for two to six weeks. The oil should turn red. Strain through a sieve and bottle. The oil heals wounds and helps prevent scarring. It is also helpful for bruises, burns, cold sores, psoriasis, sunburn, and bedsores. It makes an excellent application for the rash of shingles or chicken pox and general nerve pain. Use the oil as a rub for backache, sore muscles, and injuries to the spinal cord. It can also be made into an ointment or suppository for painful hemorrhoids or anal fissures. A lotion from the infusion can be very helpful for itchy skin conditions, especially where there is no visible rash.

### Additional Uses of St. John's Wort

In baking, a small quantity of St. John's Wort can be added to flour to improve the quality of bread. The flowers are used to produce a yellow dye and the stems a red dye. In the garden, St. John's Wort attracts bees. It does not produce nectar so few adult butterflies are attracted to it. The Grey Hairstreak Butterfly's larvae feeds on its seeds and the Gray Half-Spot Moth's larvae feeds on its foliage, making it a useful addition to a butterfly garden in regions where these Lepidoptera species are native. The flowering tops can be added to sleep pillows.

## PLANT DIETING WITH ST. JOHN'S WORT

*After choosing to diet St. John's Wort, it is time to harvest the plants and prepare your elixir. Below you will find recipes for two St. John's Wort elixirs that I made at Derrynagittah. I have described the instructions that I received from St. John's Wort for making these two elixirs. When making your own elixir you will need to listen carefully to the plants and let them guide you. See chapter 4 for more complete information on harvesting plants and preparing the elixir.*

*In advance of your plant diet it is important to prepare yourself for several days with a period of physical and spiritual purification. At Derrynagittah we make specific cleansing and dietary recommendations for each diet. You will find the recommended preparations for the St. John's Wort diet below.*

## 🌿 MAKING THE ST. JOHN'S WORT ELIXIR

You will notice that while most components in the elixir recipes below are expressed as parts of the whole, certain ingredients (notably vibrational essences, and in this instance sprigs of plant material) are listed with a specific quantity. In these cases, the amount is NOT proportional to the total amount of elixir and represents a quantity simply added to the whole. This is an intuitive, guided choice and the amount can remain the same, regardless of total quantity; that is, the same number of drops of essence can be added, whether to 20 oz. of elixir or 2 gallons.

*Elixir I*

- ❧ 3 parts infusion of flowering St. John's Wort tops
    Fresh Perforate St. John's Wort tops (made with 2 oz./60 g plant
        material per 20 fl. oz./500 ml of boiling water)
    1 sprig of Tutsan St. John's Wort
    1 sprig of Square-stemmed St. John's Wort
- ❧ 1 part tincture of Perforate St. John's Wort in mezcal
- ❧ ¼ of a part Tutsan berry infusion
- ❧ 2 drops each of Perforate and Tutsan flower essences

**Amount of elixir at diet:** Seven servings of 3 tablespoons and 1 teaspoon (50 ml) for each person

Harvesting St. John's Wort at the Summer Solstice was an experience that rapidly transported me to another world, outside of everyday time and space. I picked the flowering tops from a large St. John's Wort bed in the herb garden, which was like stepping into a sea of golden Light. I felt the familiar childlike delight and wonder of being with plants and my heart lifted, caressed and filled by their bright radiance. St. John's Wort spoke to me about the importance of boundaries and learning how to hold the suffering of others without sacrificing ourselves in the process. The lesson here is about learning not to give away a piece of our soul to others, whether partner, child, or other loved one, because if we do, we only burden them with unusable energy. The plants told me not to pity others. They reminded me to see people in need in their Divine Light. Acknowledging the light and perfection in another stimulates their radiance and encourages them to shine. I came away feeling filled with Divine presence.

*Elixir 2*

- A decoction of dried, flowering Perforate St. John's Wort (1 oz./30 g of dried plant material per 30 fl. oz./750 ml water, simmered for 10 minutes)

**Amount of elixir taken at diet:** Six servings of 4 tablespoons and 2 teaspoons (70 ml) for each person

This is an example of a simple elixir consisting solely of one ingredient, a ten minute decoction of the dried plant. In this case, the St. John's Wort had been dried after harvesting the previous summer.

## PREPARATION FOR THE ST. JOHN'S WORT DIET

### General Preparations

For three days prior to diet take NO refined sugar, added salt, meat or dairy products, strong spices, coffee, alcohol, or fermented foods. Avoid oils apart from olive oil. Do not engage in sexual activity.

### Food during the St. John's Wort Diet

For those not fasting, we recommend apples (in any form, including apple juice) and walnuts.

### Suggested Drinks

We recommend green tea, Ginger tea, Nettle tea, and hot or cold water.

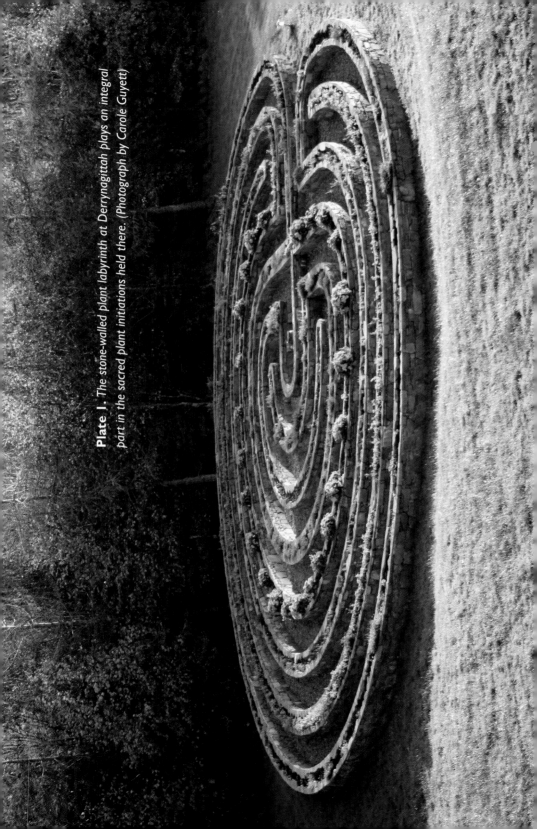

**Plate 1.** The stone-walled plant labyrinth at Derrynagittah plays an integral part in the sacred plant initiations held there. (Photograph by Carole Guyett.)

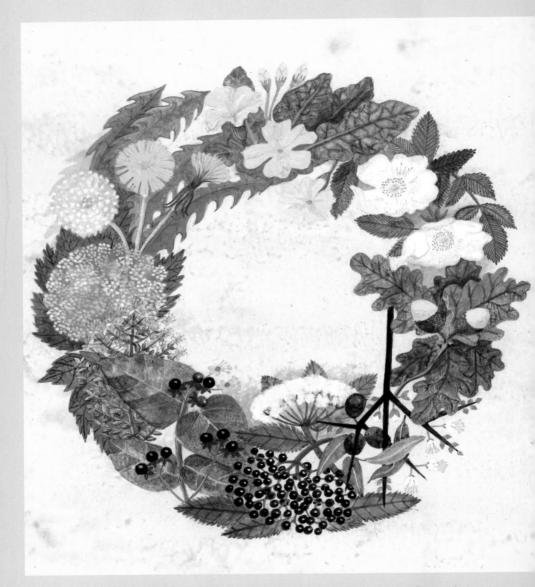

**Plate 2.** *This lovely wreath shows the eight common plants featured in the plant diets described in this book. Moving clockwise from the top, they are Primrose, Dog Rose, Oak, Blackthorn, Elder, St. John's Wort, Angelica, and Dandelion. (Illustration by Judith Evans)*

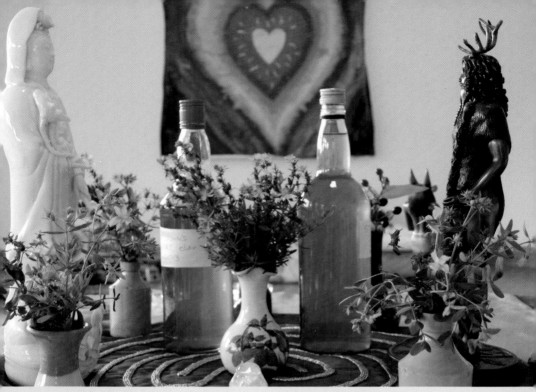

**Plate 3.** *An altar set up to honor St. John's Wort during a sacred plant initiation ceremony (Photograph by Carole Guyett)*

**Plate 4.** *Primrose in bloom (Photograph by Rowan McOnegal)*

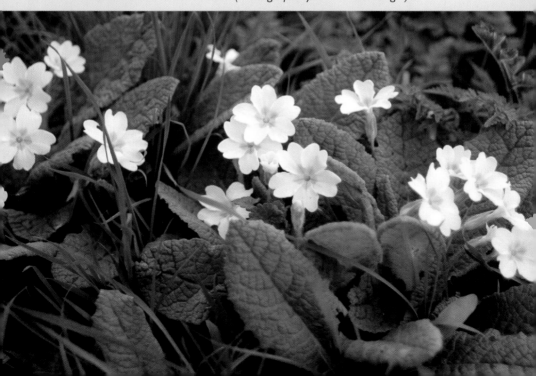

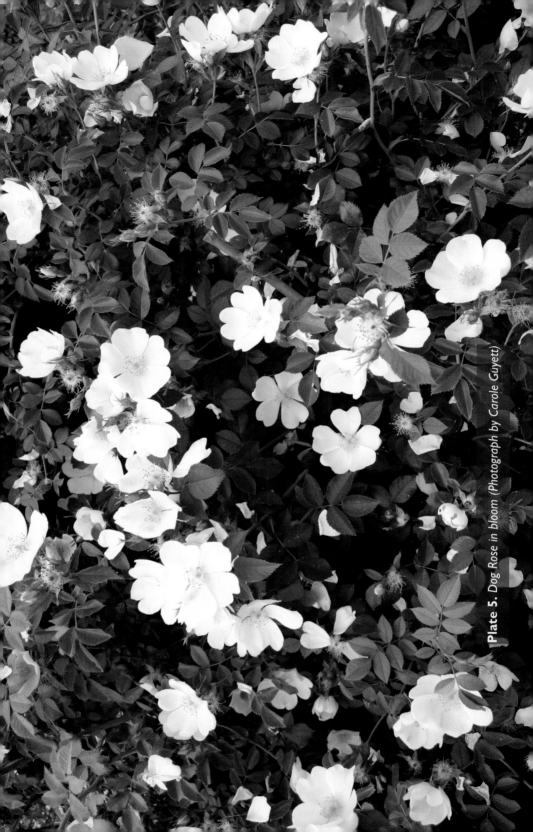

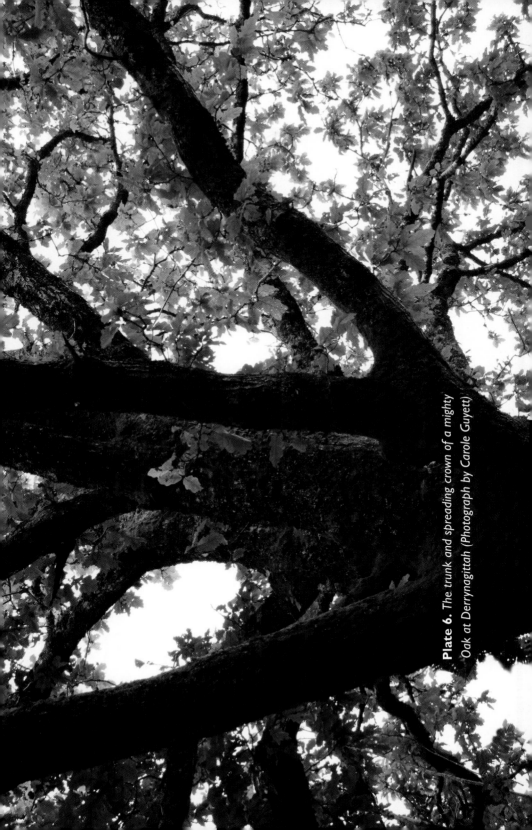

**Plate 6.** The trunk and spreading crown of a mighty Oak at Derrynagittah (Photograph by Carole Guyett)

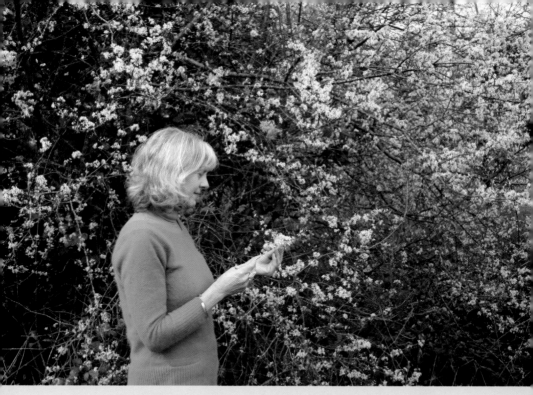

**Plate 7.** *The author and Blackthorn in early spring (Photograph by Josh Guyett)*

**Plate 8.** *Elder in bloom (Photograph by Carole Guyett)*

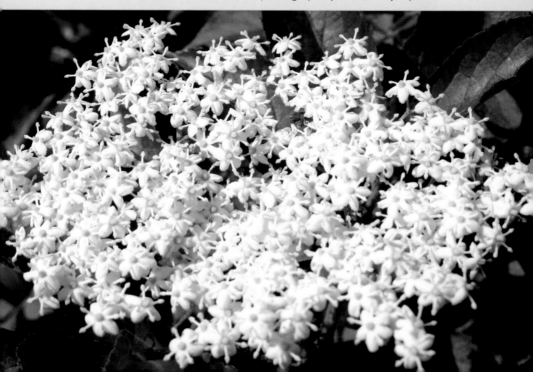

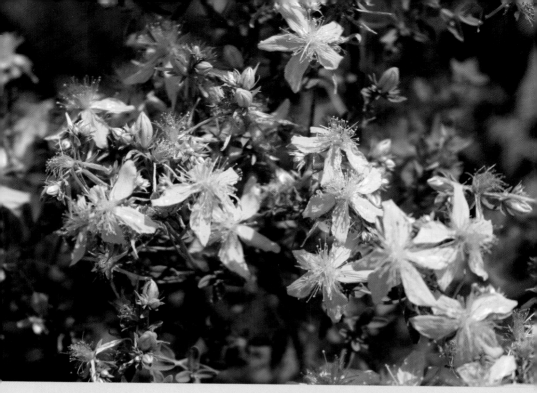

**Plate 9.** *The sunny yellow flowers of Perforate St. John's Wort (Photograph by Carole Guyett)*

**Plate 10.** *Angelica goddess. Freshly harvested Angelica roots resting on a goddess statue in the garden (Photograph by Carole Guyett)*

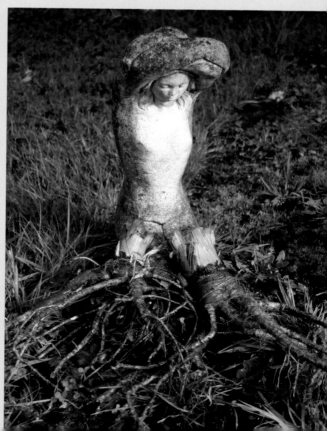

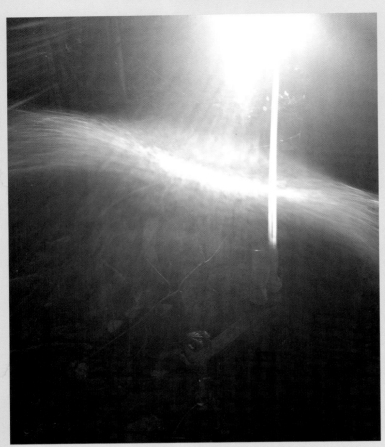

**Plate 11.** *Angelica angel. This is one of several amazing pictures taken by Erin during our Angelica plant diet. It shows what appeared to us as a magnificent being of Light carrying a light saber and pouring Divine Light over the land—perhaps Archangel Michael himself? (Photograph by Erin Summers)*

**Plate 12.** *A bowl of Dandelion flowers being infused in the sun with a small crystal skull during the making of the Dandelion Crystal Skull vibrational essence (Photograph by Carole Guyett)*

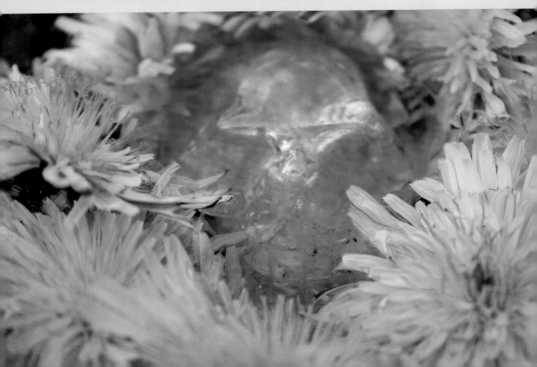

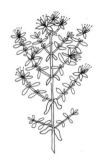

## DREAMING WITH ST. JOHN'S WORT

*Through the alchemy of sacred ceremony and by surrendering to the plant, participants in a plant diet enter into an altered state in which they form close relationships with the plant that they are dieting and receive gifts that may be physical, emotional, mental, and spiritual. Many participants gain a completely new perspective on life. The relationship with the plant is deeply transformative, facilitating access to higher consciousness, guidance, and healing. In this section people who have dieted with St. John's Wort tell the stories of their personal transformations.*

### Receiving Light

The St. John's Wort plant diets have been noteworthy for initiating experiences of Light. These experiences have taken a variety of forms for different people and this variation has been a reminder of the value of letting go of expectations, surrendering to the plant, and trusting one's individual process. There is no right or wrong experience at a plant initiation and it is neither helpful nor appropriate to compare our progress with that of others. We trust the plants, knowing they will give each of us what we need. We must simply accept what is given and do our best to learn from it. We do not know exactly what will manifest during a plant diet and we can benefit the most if we let go of trying to control our experience.

With St. John's Wort, as with any plant initiations, the effects range from subtle to intense depending on the individual. Carmel came to an initiation after receiving instructions to "turn toward the Light." She gave this account:

*I was drawn to St. John's Wort because of my sense of being drawn to the Light since the summer. I experienced some kind of shift during the summer months. I had to let go of whatever was holding me back and not to continue digging in the darkness for the way forward. I got a very clear instruction during a meditation session that I had to turn toward the Light. I felt very close to Bridget\* at this time and felt the need to be close to fire in order to light a fire in me and in others. During the week before the plant diet, I spent time connecting to the plant [in this case the Tutsan] in my own garden. This took the form of sitting with the plant or just talking to it and letting it know that I am open to receiving whatever it has to give me. What struck me during this time was the visual aspect of the plant—the specific arrangement of the green petals under the dark, red berry. The starlike arrangement appeared to me like the human form: head, arms, and legs (five petals: three big and two small). Also, the darkness of the berry struck me the whole week as a strong contrast to the luminous, yellow flower. At some stage the term* dark sun *occurred to me. Not the black sun of alchemy or Germanic mythology, but a yellow sun eclipsed by darkness that puts a black veil over it. We only see a black ball, instead of the yellow one. I felt this is the sense of depression and dark moods that cross our paths in life, like a darkness covering our Light.*

Carmel had previously attended a diet with Hawthorn that for her was extremely intense. This time, in contrast to her expectations, the plant initiation was "a very gentle experience." She explained:

*There were no new insights; no obvious emotional clearing (in contrast to the last one I did with the Hawthorn) and I found the diet itself easy. At the end I felt that I hadn't felt the Light of the plant move through my body in the way I expected. Yet I know from my own experiences with energy work and with other plant diets that intense reaction during the process is not any proof of whether it "worked." It's the subtle changes afterward looking back*

---

*Here, this participant is referring to the goddess Brigid (see chapter 12 for more on Brigid).

*on the experience that show me what has taken place. But I often go into these experiences with certain expectations, nonetheless! In the weeks after the initiation, I did feel the sense of Light subtly increase in my being. I kept meeting the plant on walks, in other people's gardens, etc. Even though I felt I hadn't really made a close connection during the diet, I can now say that it's a very definite presence in my life, an ally on my journey.*

Other initiates experienced the Light of St. John's Wort in more immediate ways. During the diet, Maura encountered "waves of diamond-light entering through the top of my head" and Maeve described "pure golden light going through my whole body." Patricia recalled, "A huge St. John's Wort flower descended upon me and I felt myself enter a kind of mystical state where I was pure Light energy. It was an incredibly beautiful experience and I think it will take me some time to integrate it." Brenda recounted, "It was as if a bright light was switched on in my head, really brilliant white light. Then I felt my whole body vibrating and golden light was pouring out of it like lots and lots of beams of sunlight coming out of me from everywhere but particularly from my heart. It felt like I was dissolving; very refreshing and cleansing." For Jennifer, St. John's Wort helped her to connect with the Light of her own life blueprint (her soul's original plan for this lifetime). During the initiation she asked for insights into her blueprint and recalled:

*St. John's Wort appeared to me as a formless being of yellowish color/light, a subtle and moving energy. St. John's Wort flew me into outer space and connected me with my blueprint and with my star energy, my star origins. It revealed that my blueprint is connected to priestess energy. The energy is calm and it balances out my emotions. I get tripped up by my emotions, my passion. My system is a little fried, overreactive, red energy, oversensitive, and inflamed. The energy of my blueprint is calming white bluish light. Accessing my blueprint connects me with dignity. It's a place where I can be fully conscious and can take action with pure intention. I connected to star energy and brought it to my lower chakras. I was tense and it felt good to open up and receive the Light.*

## Lightening the Darkness

Natasha also had the experience of receiving Light. She emphasized the compassion and gentleness of St. John's Wort and gave this account:

*I heard about the plant medicine weekend from two friends of mine and it was like a little light switch went off in me. I was particularly drawn to St. John's Wort, having taken it twenty years ago for depression while living in London. It was almost like revisiting an old friend but the experience was much, much deeper than I expected. I had to visit the story behind the past depression and look at the anger that was still holding on to me. Even though I have done a lot of inner work over the last ten years, it felt like I needed something to go even further into the source of it. St. John's Wort surprised me as I thought I might have a strong reaction to everything that had to be faced and worked through. Instead it felt like it held me, allowing me to shift through things at my own pace. I had a feeling of the plant just being so compassionate with me and supporting me on my journey, letting me take it slowly and teaching me to learn to forgive myself. I had a beautiful vision while we were journeying of connecting to the spirit of the plant. He took me on a path of light and gifted me this beautiful green light right into my heart. He gave me a crystal and said clearly to me to forgive myself and to trust in life again.*

Brenda described how the St. John's Wort had brought Light into her "inner darkness." She shared:

*During the initiation I went through different phases. Early on I felt filled with Light, very expanded and free like lots of gateways opened up to other dimensions. Then I started feeling incredibly sad, alone, abandoned, betrayed, guilty, and worthless. It was as if the St. John's Wort was shining light on all of my old stuff, starkly revealing all my issues, particularly ones I thought I had dealt with. I was nearly overwhelmed with sadness at the cruelty and grief in the world. Later on I had a beautiful dream where I received a huge amount of love and kindness and the strong message to never forget that I am loved and that I am not alone. I woke up feeling wonderful, filled with presence and a sense of ease and knowing absolutely that I am so helped and loved. I feel there has been a big cleansing, burning through and illuminating my inner darkness. I am aware of huge support and love from the St. John's Wort. My relationship with St. John's Wort has totally changed and I am very grateful.*

This cleansing effect of the Light was echoed by Yukari, who several weeks after her initiation described how St. John's Wort had cleared darkness from her. She shared, "A few years ago a fortune-teller told me that I could not live past the age of forty unless I found a way to let darkness go. It makes sense for me because I have many dark influences that I cannot let go of and the darkness has been accumulating in my mind. Since the St. John's Wort plant diet, I feel like I am cleansed."

The lightening of darkness was reiterated by Henrique, who explained how St. John's Wort had affected his subconscious mind. Some weeks after the initiation he commented:

*The St. John's Wort plant diet began some new processes inside my inner reality, like literally putting some light where before there was only darkness. When I say darkness, I mean the part that lies within myself that I'm not completely conscious of and that has the power to influence my life somehow. This "lightening the darkness within" process happened, and still happens, in a subtle and powerful way, permitting me to perceive more clearly some of the patterns that were governing some of my actions, thoughts, and emotions. Being aware of these patterns and able to make this distinction, I can start working on them, freeing myself from their negative/unconscious influence. I've been able to perceive more clearly the circles and spirals of life—patterns, emotions, and thoughts—and how deeply everything is beautifully connected. Life is beautiful, indeed. The magic of being relaxed and understanding that all my fears and problems come from inside—from my head, my mind—surely makes a huge difference in the way I deal with them. I feel free to be myself and I gave away loads of guilt that I was carrying and feeling. I realized that I was the one blaming and judging myself all the time and that kept me blocked.*

## Releasing Old Patterns

Jennifer similarly reported how St. John's Wort helped free her from old patterns:

> *On my journey to St. John's Wort, Dragonfly flew me to the house of St. John's Wort. In past journeys, I would sit around the fire in big armchairs and talk to St. John's Wort. This time the house had a glass roof and we landed on the roof. Everything on the roof was glass—the chairs, a table, and the roof itself. It was all transparent and breakable. It was very "Alice in Wonderland tea party"-esque. The spirits gathered told me to be careful because something could easily break if I stepped too hard, but they joked that nothing would fall if the glass ceiling broke because we were all spirits and could just float anyway. It seemed very much about St. John's Wort being able to transport you out of your own glass ceilings in your mind and break you out of old thought patterns and habits. It can give you a whole new way of thinking and help you to get out of the box and experience breakthroughs.*

Continuing with this theme, during the GreenBreath Jennifer uncovered

> *the belief that people can only love me because of what I do (not what I am). I was able to go to the very core of that belief in my second chakra (and my fibroids) and become pure love when I merged with St. John's Wort. Loving is about who I am and about being a Divine spirit and shining my Divine Light. I can do nothing and still I am loved and I am love.*

## Reconnecting with Nature and Spiritual Guidance

As is commonly found at plant diets, many initiates experienced a reconnection with plants and Nature. For Fernanda, this connection involved an increased awareness of her body's inner wisdom, which afterward resulted in more healthy eating. Several months after the St. John's Wort diet she recalled:

*The plant initiation was a special and beautiful experience. During the plant diet I felt like the St. John's Wort opened many doors in my mind and in my body. I felt my hair growing down into the Earth and being like roots to reconnect me with Nature in a physical way. I could feel during the ceremony a very strong reconnection with Nature and I think this starts with my body. Since the initiation my body is asking me to eat healthier food and I have completely stopped cow's milk and red meat. If I eat processed food my body doesn't accept it well. I really want to change my diet since the ceremony. It's a strong difference from before. I know this reconnection with Nature will be a step-by-step process and to eat better is definitely the first step.*

Natasha also spoke about connecting with the Earth and with our inner wisdom, describing how she particularly connected with the sound of St. John's Wort:

*I was amazed at tuning in so deeply with the St. John's Wort plants. I could hear their sounds and I wanted to sing them. Later that day Carole played the sound of a plant for us and it was the same as I had heard.\* I had this feeling of being able to hear the plants' songs and when out in the garden I felt like I could hear the vibrations of every plant I touched. It was like time just stood still and I could remember where we came from. It was a big lesson in respecting our connection to this Earth and listening to what it is telling us. It is equally important to respect, honor, and listen to our own inner knowledge and wisdom.*

## Enhancing Creativity

Many initiates reported both increased receptivity to spiritual guidance and a sense of enhanced creativity. Maura described a dream in which

---

\*At this particular plant diet I wired up a Tutsan plant to a biofeedback machine that converts signals from the plant into sound. The audio files available at audio.innertraditions.com/saplin include a track of plant music produced in this way.

*some dark Tutsan berries were placed in my womb where they firmly embedded. I saw that my womb was lit and warmed by a bright fire from below and the seeds started to germinate immediately. The day after the initiation it felt like a profound gestation was happening inside my body. It was some kind of creative process, like a dragon was stirring. Now I feel that St. John's Wort is guiding me and helping me to manifest creative ideas.*

Several weeks later Fernanda commented, "I feel like my creativity is stronger now. So many plans and dreams are popping up in my mind all the time! This has made me feel more calm about the future. I'm not as worried as I used to be about what to do. I can trust and know that the way to follow will appear for me." Carmel revealed, "I notice a much greater openness to receiving soul information since the diet. It's as if the line of communication is much clearer and the messages can flow unimpeded to and fro!"

## Anchoring New Energies on the Earth

For myself, while holding the space at the St. John's Wort diets, I felt that those who took part were blessed with new seeds to carry and were made ready for their next step, whatever that may be. There was a strong sense of collective activity for the planet and it was interesting to note that these diets attracted participants from Japan and North and South America, as well as those from all over Ireland and other parts of Europe. I'll close this chapter with my own dreaming, which illustrates St. John's Wort anchoring energies on the Earth and forming new planetary grids:

*I found myself in a dark cave with water running down the walls. There were symbols and cave paintings of hands, which came to life and started moving. Then I saw a large St. John's Wort flower and I was sucked into a tunnel in the center of the flower. Next I came up in what appeared to be a crop circle in a field of St. John's Wort. It was a valley and the entire area was covered in St. John's Wort in bloom, quite stunning. I realized I was walking the edges of some sort of design that seemed to be made up of flowers with six petals. I knew it was St. John's Wort, but my mind was saying, "How*

*can this be St. John's Wort when it has too many petals?" I heard the St.*
*John's Wort laughing at me and saying, "You cannot be serious! Let it go."*
*I kept walking and realized that this was the flower of life design (a well-*
*known symbol from sacred geometry) and that I was supposed to walk it as*
*a circuit. Knowing the design, my mind thought this was an enormous task*
*and I heard myself say, "No, you cannot be serious!" As I walked further, I*
*started to feel dizzy, disorientated, and nauseous. Then I became anxious;*
*worried that I would vomit in this beautiful place. Again, I was aware of*
*the St. John's Wort laughing at me; not in an unkind way, just helping me*
*see how ridiculous my thoughts were and not to take myself so seriously.*
*Suddenly the whole scene started to spin and I was caught in a blur. Then*
*the flower of life was in 3-D. It was transposed to the top of the labyrinth at*
*Derrynagittah and there were three levels and many different colors. The*
*colors were merging and bleeding into each other, mixing and flowing. It's*
*hard to put into words, but it seemed that different realities were mixing*
*together. Then I was high above myself and watching as the labyrinth/flower*
*of life uncurled itself like a strand of DNA uncoiling. It was at the same time*
*like a strip of video film unwinding, quite beautiful and intriguing to watch.*
*It moved outward over the land and then across the planet, encircling it and*
*wrapping it like a bandage, going round and round. This coil was anchoring*
*new energies and forming new grids around the Earth—beautiful geometric*
*forms that pulsated with frequencies of pure love, grace, beauty, and peace,*
*each with their own color and sound and coming together like an amazing*
*symphony of Light. It was exquisite.*

I know from experience that if a dreaming like this comes, it is a message
that needs to be acted upon. There is no value in receiving far-out dreams
or visions if they do not serve a concrete purpose in real life. What's more,
I have a responsibility to use what is given in the best way I can. Anything
less is disrespectful and dishonoring both to Spirit and myself. I have to
be careful not to simply enjoy the awesome experience and move on without it changing anything. That would simply be more consumerism and
reflect a serious lack of appreciation. Regarding this particular dreaming:
at this point in time I cannot say I have fully understood or acted upon

it, but its impact has stayed with me and I know it is part of an unfolding process that is gradually teaching me more about the plants and how I can best serve both them and the planet, including how best to work with the labyrinth. A tangible, material effect has been that the dream reminded me of the significance of the Flower of Life design—something I have worked with inconsistently over the years (see page 107). It was a clear call both for me to work with the symbol more consciously and to include it in this book. This beautiful image can be extremely beneficial for meditation and other purposes.

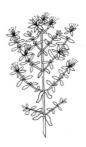

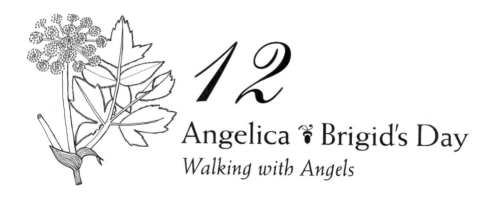

# 12
## Angelica ❦ Brigid's Day
### *Walking with Angels*

K nown as the herb of angels and said to enable one to commune with the angelic realm, the magnificent and stately Angelica has been respected and esteemed as a medicine since ancient times. Reputed to cure almost any malady from plague to tuberculosis, Angelica stands tall and graceful, a royal messenger from Spirit, the queen whose globe-shaped flowers are her crowning glory. Angelica connects with Spirit and carries the protection of angels and archangels, holding sovereignty with unashamed self-expression and beauty. Ruled by the sun and carrying Fire, she grounds celestial energies through her strong central column and is said to have been grown in the gardens of Atlantis.* Traditionally ascribed as male and associated with the astrological sign of Leo, she can also be very feminine, revealing her connection with Venus (see color plate 10).

---

*According to Greek philosopher Plato (429–347 B.C.E.), Atlantis was a pre-Egyptian civilization with an advanced technology, based on silica and crystals, that provided an abundant source of power. Many people view Atlantis as a symbol of harmonious civilization and consider the Atlantean era to have been an important age in human development, where great emphasis was given to healing, meditation, and the development of consciousness. The Atlantean civilization destroyed itself by using its technology for unwholesome purposes. There is said to have been a major cataclysm in which the land was swallowed up by the sea. Some consider Hy-Brasil (a mythical land located in the Atlantic Ocean off the west coast of Ireland) to be a part of the remnants of Atlantis.

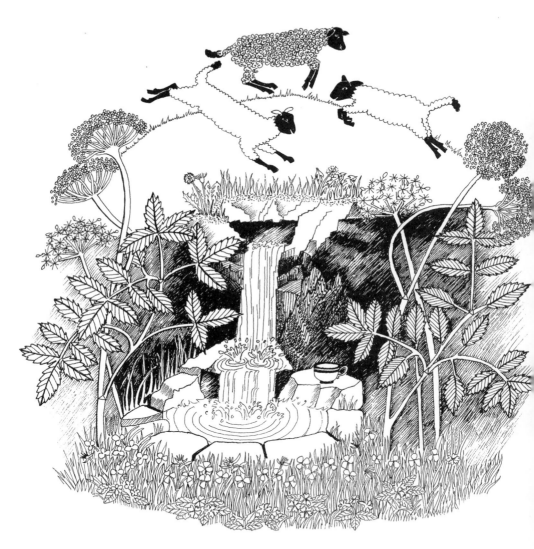

Brigid's Day, or Imbolc, marks the beginning of spring as seeds stir
in the ground and sap begins to rise.

Along with Angelica's pungent scent and taste comes the potent presence of Archangel Michael, the masculine chief of the angelic realms. Michael represents the all-encompassing strength and protection of the Divine. Though he was known to the ancient Hebrews and described in the Bible, the forerunners of the Celts honored him as their supreme masculine guardian long before the birth of Abraham. Equipped with his golden shield and sword of truth he is ready to attend to anyone who calls for protection. He lends support, courage, confidence, and the knowledge that anything is possible.

Carrying the fiery qualities of illumination and inspiration, Angelica is closely linked to Brigid's Day and the creativity of spring. This is a plant of renewal and strong life-force energy. Angelica activates and strengthens our inner fire and is a perfect plant to diet with at this time.

## BRIGID'S DAY—IMBOLC
### *Renewal of the Life Force*

In contemporary Ireland, this festival is known as Brigid's Day. It is celebrated on February 1 and marks the beginning of spring. Other names for this holiday are Candlemas and Oimealg, traditionally celebrated on the night of January 31. This is the festival of the Celtic Goddess Brigid, daughter of the Daghdha, Father God of the Tuatha De Danaan. Brigid (also known as Bride and Brid) is the Goddess in her maiden aspect. She is the Keeper of the Sacred Flame and the Holy Wells; Goddess of Poetry, Smithcraft, and Healing. She brings creative inspiration and is associated with fertility, midwifery, Fire, and Water.

At Imbolc in temperate lands, the seeds are stirring in the ground, sap is rising, buds are forming, and bulbs are pushing through the soil. As the days lengthen, there is an urge to wake up and move forward, bringing through the visions and dreams that have been nurtured over the winter.

In Ireland, tradition has it that Brigid visited homes on Brigid's Eve and people would leave food and drink (especially milk) on windowsills and doorsteps in order to nourish her and receive her blessings as she passed by. It was customary (and still is in some areas) to leave a cloth (*brat Bhride* or Brigid's mantle) outside on a windowsill, fence, or tree branch so that Brigid would bless the cloth and bring the power of healing and protection. This could then be cut into pieces and shared with others, to be used for fertility and for curing illness throughout the year. Another enduring tradition is to make Brigid's crosses from rushes or other grasses. These are hung over the entrance to the house or in the kitchen to ensure protection and prosperity in the coming year. People also made Brideogs (Brigid's dolls) from grasses. These dolls represent the Goddess, bringing fertility and good fortune. One tradition is to give your dreams and intentions to the Brideog and release her into a river or other living body of water.

This is a time for spring cleaning and to celebrate the renewal of life force. Connect with the seeds stirring in the dark soil, feel the seeds within yourself. What is preparing to sprout and grow? Consider and feed the ideas and dreams that you have cultivated over the winter, making preparations for these to emerge. The Goddess Brigid is now a national saint

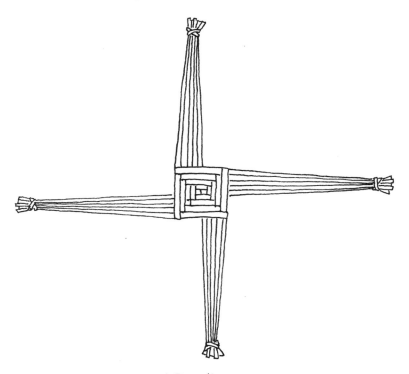

*A Brigid's cross*

and in modern Ireland numerous sites are dedicated to her, especially holy wells. In Kildare, the Brigidine nuns keep alight her perpetual flame.

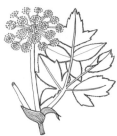

## ANGELICA—THE HERB OF ANGELS
*Angelica archangelica: Garden Angelica*
**Plant family:** Umbelliferae (Carrot Family).

**Other common names:** Garden Angelica; Masterwort; Archangel; The Angel's Herb; Bellyache Root; Root of the Holy Ghost; Herba Angelica (Angel's Plant); Norwegian Angelica; *Bliúcán* (Irish—usually refers to Wild Angelica).

**Description:** Angelica is a tall, striking plant, usually biennial, growing up to nine or ten feet in height. It has green hollow stems, large leaves made up of smaller leaflets in groups of three, and bears umbels of greenish white flowers typically in May and June of its second year. The whole plant is highly aromatic.

**Habitat:** It likes damp places and is cultivated in gardens. It is also naturalized in parts of Europe, often found near bodies of water. Angelica readily self-seeds and is best propagated by seeds sown as soon as it is ripe, in August or September. Planting Nettles as a companion plant can increase the yield of Angelica oil by as much as 80 percent.

**Distribution:** Garden Angelica is native to northern Europe, Russia, Iceland, Greenland, and the Himalayas. It is widely cultivated and has been introduced to many northern temperate regions. Several species of Angelica are native to North America, the most valuable medicinally being American Angelica (*Angelica atropurpurea*), found on the East Coast from Newfoundland to Delaware and West Virginia, and west to Illinois and Wisconsin.

**Species:** Wild Angelica (*Angelica sylvestris*), with its pink/purple furrowed stems and red-tinged white or pink flowers, grows throughout Europe and is closely related to Garden Angelica. It can be used interchangeably and is considered a gentler version. In North America, the native purple-stemmed *Angelica atropurpurea* (known as Purple or

American Angelica) is the most commonly used for medicine and has similar properties to Garden Angelica, which is cultivated in some areas. Chinese Angelica (*Angelica sinensis*) is a native of East Asia and has different medicinal actions.

**Parts used:** Root and rhizome should be harvested in autumn of the first year before the first frosts. Seeds can be gathered by cutting the ripe seed heads in July or August. Leaves and fresh young stems are to be picked in May or June, preferably before flowering. When harvesting in the wild, be careful NOT to confuse Angelica with Hemlock, which is extremely poisonous.

## Angelica as a Spirit Medicine

As reflected in its flower essence, the spirit of Angelica offers the experience of protection and guidance from spiritual beings. It connects with the angelic realm and particularly brings in the energies of Archangel Michael. However or whatever you perceive him to be, this energy brings a major influx of Light with strength, guardianship, and purification. This is Fire energy, with a potency that can cut through and transform anything, cleansing and purifying, clearing negativity and reconsecrating that which has been defiled. Sovereignty is restored and with it feelings of safety, strength, and confidence.

Angelica carries profound protection to soothe, support, and reassure even the most vulnerable. This is not an imagined protection of the mind. This is real embodied protection with palpable effects. There is enormous healing and strengthening in the flames of Angelica, a spiritual Light, which pours down through the central column of the body, targeting wherever it is needed. Angelica not only purifies and protects, it helps us return to that place of the still, shining lake within. We know our connection to Earth and Sky and we experience the presence of Spirit within and without. We know that we are never alone and that all is well.

It is not only Archangel Michael who comes forward with Angelica. At times it can be as if an entire heavenly host has come forth. This is an amazing plant for establishing connections with all kinds of spirit beings and alternate realities. It can bring through an awareness of ancient civilizations and has a specific connection with Atlantis.

The fiery Angelica spirit also helps us awaken and rekindle our own fires, activating passion, willpower, and creativity. It helps us open ourselves to receive inspiration and information from Spirit. When Angelica comes to you it can bring guidance at the time and it can give notice that you will soon receive messages, visions, or creative ideas from the invisible realm. By putting us in touch with our higher self, Angelica assists us in knowing who we are and why we are here. It fills us with radiant Light energy, helping us to connect with our highest and best purpose.

The ability to travel to other realms is facilitated by smoking dried Angelica leaves. This smoke can also be used as a smudge for the purification of a place or a person. It combines well with Rosemary and Frankincense to cleanse a temple space before or after ceremony. Dried Angelica leaves also make a helpful addition to a healing incense. An infusion of Angelica can similarly be used as a wash for surfaces, windows, and so forth to purify the atmosphere in a house or temple. To place a protective seal, the infusion can be sprinkled around the boundaries of a plot or at the four corners of a house. The infusion may be added to a bath to clear negativity and to soothe, strengthen, and heal the spirit. For spiritual healing it is highly beneficial to soak in a bath containing Angelica infusion or fresh Angelica leaves and flowers. Angelica oil is utilized for anointing and the dried root is carried as a protective amulet. Angelica is used to communicate with or invoke Archangel Michael or others from the angelic realm. It is also employed to connect with Atlantis and can be used to invoke the element of Fire and the direction of the South. As a bringer of Light, Angelica is associated with Brigid's Day and the returning light of the spring. It is also linked with the peaking of the sun's light at the Summer Solstice.

## Angelica as a Flower Essence

**Key words to describe this essence:**
Spiritual guidance and protection; connection with angels.

Angelica essence brings feelings of protection and guidance from spiritual beings. It helps us build a relationship with our higher self and with the spiritual world in general. It is especially helpful for those who feel disconnected or cut off from spiritual guidance and protection. Angelica encourages a tangible, living relationship with the angelic realm and assists during threshold experiences such as giving birth, dying, festival celebrations, and other ceremonial work.

## Angelica in Folklore and History

This remarkable plant has a long history of use as a protective herb against infection and illness as well as all evil and enchantments. It is universally known by its botanical name, which derives from the Greek *angelos* meaning "a spiritual messenger." In Pagan Europe it was dedicated to deities of the sun, and with the coming of Christianity, the plant became linked with the angelic realm. It was especially associated with Archangel Michael, and it is seen to bloom around his feast day, May 8. It was also connected with the Annunciation, which falls close to the Spring Equinox. Archangel Michael is credited with bringing Angelica to the attention of humans, as he is said to have appeared in a dream to a fourteenth-century monk or physician and revealed the plant's ability to cure plague. His instructions were to hold a piece of root in the mouth to drive away the "pestilentiall aire." Angelica soon emerged as a prime remedy for the bubonic plague that was rife in Europe at the time. The plant became one of the great medicinal herbs of the Middle Ages, used to treat an impressive range of conditions. When European colonists arrived in North America, they discovered many Indian tribes using American Angelica in the same way that their own healers used the European species, particularly for respiratory ailments and tuberculosis.

Angelica's protection was widely sought in medieval Europe. The root was carried to protect from malevolent energies, it was added to bath water to remove curses or spells, and the powdered root was sprinkled around the home to avert evil influences. Used as an antidote for harmful potions, Angelica was taken to remedy the adverse effects of alcohol and extended to the treatment of alcoholism as well.

## Angelica in Contemporary Herbal Medicine

Angelica has great powers as a warming and stimulating tonic. It brings Fire to the body, improving and normalizing physiological function, especially in cold, damp conditions. A hot tea helps resolve colds and flu, with the seeds being particularly diaphoretic and helpful for fevers when combined with Yarrow. Antibacterial and antifungal, the whole plant is useful in epidemics, protecting against infection. It defends and sustains the heart and circulation while comforting the spirits. As a warming and stimulating expectorant, Angelica is beneficial for a variety of lung conditions including asthma, bronchitis, bronchial catarrh, and pneumonia. In practice I mainly use the tinctured root, although root, leaves, young stems, and seeds can all be made into tea or tincture.

Angelica is also an aromatic bitter and gastric stimulant, strengthening and enhancing digestion, improving appetite, and relieving nausea and indigestion, especially when associated with low stomach acid. Antispasmodic and carminative, it helps relieve wind and spasm, warming and invigorating stomach, intestines, liver, and spleen. As a circulatory tonic, long-term use of Angelica improves the health of the vascular system and makes a good general tonic for elderly people. The plant can help in Raynaud's disease (a circulatory disorder in which there is an exaggerated response to cold, causing white, numb fingers, toes, ears, and nose) and has a reputation for treating arteriosclerosis (thickening and hardening of the arteries). Angelica is also an effective women's tonic, warming and stimulating pelvic circulation, toning the uterus, and regulating the menstrual cycle. It relieves menstrual cramps and can be useful as part of a treatment for pelvic inflammatory disease. To be avoided in pregnancy due to its stimulation of the womb, in childbirth it can be used to help expel a retained placenta.

The stimulating tonic effects of Angelica extend to the nervous system and are beneficial for nervous exhaustion and chronic fatigue. It is also used to treat urinary tract conditions as well as rheumatism and arthritis. Regular use of the tea causes an aversion to alcohol and is used in treatment for alcoholism. Care should be taken in cases of peptic ulceration or inflammation since Angelica's heat and stimulation may be unsuitable for these conditions.

Externally, an infusion can be used as an eyebath for sore eyes and also makes a skin lotion for wounds, scabies, itching, and neuralgia. A tea or the powdered root can be applied to old ulcers to clean and heal them. The fresh leaves are used in compresses for inflammations, pleurisy, and bronchitis.

### Additional Uses of Angelica

The young stalks are candied and used for decorating cakes and puddings. They are also used to sweeten stewed rhubarb and orange marmalade and can be cooked as a vegetable like celery or peeled and added to salads. The leaves are eaten as a vegetable in Greenland and Scandinavia. The oil is used in aromatherapy and perfumery.

Angelica root is a constituent of the famous *Eau de Melisse des Carmes*, or Carmelite Water, an elixir originally distilled by nuns for their king as a revitalizing and uplifting aromatic tonic. Angelica is an ingredient in Swedish bitters* and is used in a number of varieties of cordial, wine, vodka, gin, and liqueurs such as Benedictine and Chartreuse.

## PLANT DIETING WITH ANGELICA

*After choosing to diet Angelica, it is time to harvest the plants and prepare your elixir. Below you will find recipes for two Angelica elixirs, one that I made for a ceremonial plant diet at Derrynagittah and another that I made for a plant diet at Sweetwater Sanctuary in Vermont. I have described the instructions that I received from Angelica for making these two elixirs. When making your own elixir you will need to listen carefully to the plants and let them guide you. See chapter 4 for more complete information on harvesting plants and preparing the elixir.*

*In advance of your plant diet it is important to prepare yourself for several days with a period of physical and spiritual purification. At Derrynagittah we make specific cleansing and dietary recommendations for each diet. You will find the recommended preparations for the Angelica diet below.*

---

*Swedish bitters are an herbal tonic said to have been formulated by Paracelsus in the sixteenth century and popularized more recently by Austrian herbalist Maria Treben.

## 🌿 MAKING THE ANGELICA ELIXIR

You will notice that while most components in the elixir recipes below are expressed as parts of the whole, certain ingredients (notably vibrational essences) are listed with a specific quantity. In these cases, the amount is NOT proportional to the total amount of elixir and represents a quantity simply added to the whole. This is an intuitive, guided choice and the amount can remain the same, regardless of total quantity; that is, the same number of drops of essence can be added, whether to 20 oz. of elixir or 2 gallons.

*Elixir I*

- ❧ I part tincture of Angelica stems, flowers, and leaves and I teaspoon Fennel seeds in Poire William*
- ❧ ½ part Angelica seed tincture in Poire William
- ❧ I part Angelica root tincture in vodka
- ❧ 2½ parts Angelica aromatic water
- ❧ ¹⁄₁₀ of a part Carmelite water†

**Amount of elixir taken at diet:** Six servings of 2 tablespoons and 2 teaspoons (40 ml) for each person

Pears were a strong feature of this elixir. I still do not mentally understand the connection between Pears and Angelica, but a strong feeling drove me to visit Galway City in quest of a pear-flavored spirit I could use in the making of the elixir. The fact that when I found something suitable it was called *Eau de Vie* (Water of Life) was a bonus as far as I was concerned. There was an outstanding sense of beauty in every step of making this elixir. Not only did the ingredients smell heavenly and literally make my mouth water (typical of a bitter herb), there was also a wonderful sense of angelic presence. As I sat with the Angelica, preparing to harvest her delights, I called to Spirit and the entire area was imbued with a magnificent presence, identified by me as both Raphael (the great Archangel of Healing) and Michael. I played my xylophone

---

*Poire William is a pear-flavored *Eau de Vie,* a commercial spirit made in France and available online in a range of flavors. I used this to make the Angelica tincture.
†Carmelite water is distilled from Angelica root, Lemon Balm, Lemon rind, Cinnamon, Cloves, Nutmeg, and Coriander. It is available for purchase online.

through the plant's wheels of light (plants have energy centers just as we do) and, feeling the notes resonate in my own body, I found myself in the center of her reddish-green stem, traveling with a radiant Light. Much later, while stirring together the elixir in its final stages of preparation, I felt a ring of huge and magnificent beings around the pot, giving support and blessings. I stopped for a moment, quite taken aback, and they instructed me to "just keep stirring," saying they would add blessings as I stirred. A profound feeling of peace descended and I felt a deep sense that all was well. "We are with you," they told me, "there is nothing to worry about."

### Elixir 2

- ⅒ of a part pear juice from canned home-grown pears
- 2 parts infusion of dried Angelica root
- I part tincture of fresh Angelica root in brandy
- ½ of a part infusion of fresh Angelica seeds in white wine
- I part infusion of Angelica leaves and flowers
- 7 drops Angelica flower essence

**Amount of elixir taken at diet:** Seven servings of 2 tablespoons and 2 teaspoons (40 ml) for each person

This elixir was for a plant diet I ran at Sweetwater Sanctuary in Vermont, the home of my dear friend Pam Montgomery. It was a plant initiation for some of Pam's advanced students who were keen to participate in as much of the process as possible. Pam had harvested and prepared the various ingredients prior to my arrival from Ireland and we performed the final mixing ceremony as a group on the first day. It was such a delight and privilege to share this sacred alchemy with a gathering of enthusiastic and like-minded plant lovers!

##  PREPARATION FOR THE ANGELICA PLANT DIET

### General Preparations

For three days prior to the diet take NO refined sugar, added salt, meat or dairy products, strong spices, coffee, alcohol, or fermented foods. Avoid oils apart from olive oil. Do not engage in sexual activity.

*Food during the Angelica Diet*
For those not fasting we recommend almonds, pears, honey.

*Suggested Drinks*
We recommend Fennel or Ginger teas and hot or cold water.

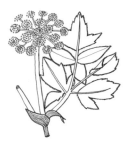

## DREAMING WITH ANGELICA

*Through the alchemy of sacred ceremony and by surrendering to the plant, participants in a plant diet enter into an altered state in which they form close relationships with the plant that they are dieting and receive gifts that may be physical, emotional, mental, and spiritual. Many participants gain a completely new perspective on life. The relationship with the plant is deeply transformative, facilitating access to higher consciousness, guidance, and healing. In this section people who have dieted with Angelica tell the stories of their personal transformations.*

### Winged Ones and Angels
Powerful energies emerged at the Angelica diets, described by Amanda as "the gentle within the primordial." She went on to say, "I felt a strong connection to the Angelic realm itself, but within that strong fiery primordial energy there was gentleness and lightness." Numerous participants described encountering angels, primarily Archangel Michael as well as Gabriel (famous messenger who inspires artists and communicators), Raphael, and Uriel (Archangel of Wisdom and Light) to name but a few. April recalled:

*Bending over us were gigantic angelic figures, tending us all like so many small plants in a garden. I also saw these beings shaping DNA: great huge*

*spirals that only became tiny upon entering our human cells. Returning*
*from this journey I was given a message that I could develop the ability*
*to perceive, behind my fellow humans, the angelic beings who guide and*
*support us and suffuse us with Light. Since then, when I've had feelings*
*of resentment or jealousy toward someone, I can conjure the image of the*
*huge guardian angel who tends that person so lovingly. How could my*
*heart not be softened?*

At our ceremonies the winged ones were present in all their forms. This is Pam's account after drinking the elixir for the first time:

*As I sat by the stream taking in the essence of Angelica, my senses shifted*
*into heightened awareness as an exquisite scene of winged ones (birds)*
*displayed an array of acrobatics, stream bathing, and song before my eyes.*
*I sat transfixed by what I was observing. How could I have missed this*
*before? Surely these birds had done this very same thing many times and*
*yet in all my years of sitting in this same spot, I had never observed life and*
*all of its happenings in quite this way. I felt in that moment that I was being*
*prepared for a slice of life that perhaps I had never experienced before.*

## A Portal to the Upper Worlds

Sal described how Angelica consistently took her to the "as above," saying:

*In every journey I experienced with Angelica there were always common*
*threads. She would continually offer a portal to the angelic realms or*
*upper worlds. We were surrounded by effervescent white Light and she*
*blew white Light, life-force energy, into my heart and it traveled in waves*
*out into my whole being. She told me this symbolized purity and connection*
*to Source energy, to the Divine. This was also symbolic of the healing she*
*could offer to people with heart problems.*

The connection to the Heavens was a common experience with initiates recalling "visiting different galaxies," "traveling to Sirius," and "going to some other place in the Cosmos." Several months after the diet, Dee recounted how her experience of the Heavens had awakened an interest in astrology. "Since the Angelica initiation I have become very interested in astrology, in an intuitive way. Angelica took me on a journey into the above direction, the Heavens and the solar system. I felt and heard the planets spin within and since then it's as if the healing love of the above world has come alive and lives inside of me."

For many, Angelica carried a strong energy of the Divine Feminine and the Goddess. Amanda's experience gave her a new appreciation of the plant world:

*Angelica is a very potent and true gift of the Goddess and the sacred feminine. Angelica showed me how the Goddess will call forth specific plants as sweet medicine at very specific times to help us. Angelica is a key messenger of the Age of Flowers, bringing hope, comfort, healing, and connection. This gave me a whole new appreciation for the flowers and plants and again I was shown how each of these plants is a key, dynamic, and irreplaceable being on the web.*

For Dee, the sacred feminine brought ancestral healing. She shared afterward:

*Angelica has infused me deeply with the blessings of the Divine Feminine. This blessed plant spirit has assisted the healing of trauma in my mother lines in my ancestral lineage. Many of the deeply ingrained patterns within me that were not serving are transforming. Many of these related issues that once greatly concerned me no longer dominate my consciousness.*

## Light of Healing and Transformation

People reported healing experiences on many levels. Mary told later how the Angelica initiation

*was such an incredible experience and most definitely changed my life. Working with Angelica was like having a spotlight shine on your life and you could see behind your shadows and around the corners. There was no place to hide. Now I'm more able to see how my thoughts really do create my life. One of the gifts I received while journeying with Angelica was a paintbrush with which she told me I could paint my life however I wished. Another profound experience was the GreenBreath during which I was able to release rage that I'd been holding on to for so long I can't remember where or when it started.*

April, a healer, described how the Angelica inspired a development in her practice:

*Three days after the initiation, I had a powerful dream in which I was shown the hospital of the future. It was a round or maybe twelve-sided building with a light-filled central courtyard. Here the patient would stand under the sky and receive the down pouring of heavenly healing energy. Around the courtyard were a series of treatment rooms for the removal of specific energy blockages. So one would go into one of the rooms, work with a practitioner to open one's channels, then step into the courtyard to receive the healing energy. The feeling of the descending healing Light was very much like the spirit presence of Angelica. Now when I do reflexology treatments or practice plant spirit healing, I call on Angelica to assist us (both myself and the client) in opening to that lovely healing energy.*

## Compassion and Connection

An outstanding feature of these initiations was the amount of love, comfort, and care experienced. For me, the air in the temple was thick with magnificent beings emanating profound compassion and this sense of being loved and cared for was reiterated time and time again. Amanda described the messages from Angelica as being "about connection and not feeling alone; about the sacred law that love is all there is; about comfort and care." She went on to say how challenging this experience was for her, how it highlighted her own difficulty to receive love and to love herself:

*I kept hearing the words, "The reflection we offer is not harsh." On the whole however, these messages of love and comfort, connection and positive reflection were actually quite difficult for me to hear, as they struck a core wounded place or bitterness within me. So I spent the entire ceremony simply trying to be able to receive those messages from Angelica without resistance. I was also seeking to mend that place within my own sacred masculine that can't receive the amazing blessings and messages of this plant that is really about love, comfort, and being seen and held in one's sacred essence. The first few doses I took just knocked me out completely. I either would fall asleep right away or get so relaxed that I would need to lie down, half asleep. It was only on the second day that I was able to take a dose and stay awake. I feel as if by going to sleep and into the dream it helped me get out of the mind maze. In one of my half-asleep moments I felt myself suddenly warm, relaxed, held, feeling light, and loved. All these colors were swirling around me, like liquid golds, pinks, and blues. I heard, "You only know a sliver of what you really are." Angelica truly wishes us to embrace that which we already are instead of always striving to be different. One of the biggest issues though, for many people, is loneliness. When working with Angelica, I really had to address the issue of my loneliness. I see my loneliness and living alone, single and without a partner, as a constant reflection of both rejecting and being rejected. I need to allow a shift in reflection so that I realize I'm not alone. Angelica said, "I am love. I am always with you."*

April also received a strong message about love and how we are never alone or separate, in this instance referring particularly to birth and death. Angelica provided her with tangible ways of helping others in the process of passing over. She gave this beautiful account:

*During another vision journey, we were guided to receive a gift from the Angelica spirit. Mine was a small nest of downy white feathers, which fit into the palm of my hand. Along with the gift came a whole series of images concerning birth and death—the passing into and out of human form. Beings of Light were co-creating a "nest" of Light and matter for the incarnating soul to inhabit and then, at the end of life, they made a matrix of pure Light to receive the Light-body of the one who had just died. I was invited to bring Angelica to my side and into my hands to help in making these spirit nests when I'm in the presence of birth or death. A few days after the Angelica initiation, I dreamed of gathering white feathers that were growing on plants. The next day, I found some downy goose feathers in grasses along the road where I walk (some geese live on a nearby farm), so I brought home a pocketful of feathers. Then I dreamed of putting white feathers into envelopes to mail them off to people. Was this a hint to try to spread the messages of the plants? A few weeks later, my brother-in-law died. On my altar I made a tiny shrine for him—a candle surrounded by a nest of white feathers—and I visualized his spirit being received in that gentle, illumined place shown to me by Angelica. When I wrote to his wife and daughters, I breathed Angelica into the envelope, asking her to accompany my words. There was a message I heard repeatedly during the days of the Angelica initiation, "no separateness, no time." Though I'm not yet sure of all the implications of these words, I know they are comforting when applied to the relationship between the living and the departed. We're not really so separated as things might appear. Time does not have all that much relevance.*

Several months later, she went on to say,

*In the year since the initiation, sadly, several friends have died and for each I have beseeched that Light-filled Angelica spirit being to guide their journeys into the next realm. Sitting in the presence of the dying, I have felt Angelica's love and radiance fill the room, offering consolation as well as assurance that the departing one is guided, protected, and deeply blessed. When I want to find within myself that ephemeral bridge connecting me to loved ones who have died, I ask for help from Angelica and it seems as if the filaments of that bridge are illumined for me.*

## Healing Self-Concept and Remembering Who You Are

Maura related, "Angelica helps heal a damaged self-concept." This was echoed by Lindsey, who described how Angelica's Light had dispelled an old and outworn concept of herself:

*For me, this has been profound in helping move the grief and guilt that I carry. That is the essence, for me, of Angelica's amazing presence and healing power; it is in her Light. She shines new light on everything and in doing so instantly provides another way to see, understand, and visualize things. Angelica helps shift mental images that hold negative patterns of self-concept by shining new light that dispels fear, shame, fragmentation, guilt, anger, and dis-ease, allowing for the foundational energetic imprint to shift.*

Similarly, Mary said that since the Angelica initiation she views herself differently. "Because of this experience with Angelica I see myself with more clarity—the good, the bad, and the ugly—and I can look at myself with compassion and acceptance. I don't have to beat myself up for not being enough, for not being perfect." Sal was encouraged on her life path and urged to trust:

*Angelica showed me profound visions of me teaching; teaching both adults and children the magic and beauty of the plants. I know this is truth. I know that a huge part of my life purpose is to share the Divine wisdom of Mother Earth. I was downloaded strongly with remembrance, with the cellular memory of my ancestors. She showed me a white crystal Light path and indicated to me that my direction is looked after. I will be guided. I will be shown the way . . . to trust.*

## Freeing the Heart, Choosing Joy

For many there was an emphasis on the heart. Linda spoke of the enormous amount of love and heat she felt in her heart and Naira said, "I was feeling and seeing through my heart." Brenda recalled that the Angelica seemed to "pierce" her heart and she was startled by traveling so deep within it. She explains:

*My ego was disappointed to find pain and grief in my heart. I was thinking, "What's wrong with me? Why am I heartbroken again?" But the Angelica told me it's okay to feel like this, to let myself feel the pain and release it. The Angelica said this is helpful, not weakness or self-indulgence. She said that if pain is stored in the heart then it has to be released and the ability to feel is a great gift. The Angelica went in with strong green energy and cleared another layer out of my heart. I was told that the pain is not all mine, that some of this feeling is for the collective. Now my heart feels like it's been ripped open. Last night Anne was describing her husband's bypass surgery and how they broke the bones of his chest in order to get at his heart and then had to wire it up again afterward. That image keeps coming back to me and my heart feels really soft and vulnerable. I can see the emerald light in my heart space. It's good, even though I want to cry all the time. The Angelica is helping me to feel the pain and let it flow through. I was also told that I can choose joy instead of suffering. It may sound contradictory but it's just a choice and there was a sense of complete love and acceptance of whatever is chosen. They said suffering is not needed to create spiritual growth and there are other ways to become aware of who you truly are. We have become used to suffering on Earth, but we are now on the brink of a collective change and different ways of learning will emerge for humans. We don't need to hold pain in our hearts.*

### Releasing Pain

Several people experienced physical discomfort at these diets including aches and pains, nausea and vomiting. Naira described how she "felt very exhausted with a headache and needed to lie down," while Brenda reported that she felt "really ill." Linda said she was "sore as anything," yet "despite the aches and pains it was so beautiful." Some initiates interpreted their symptoms as the release of tissue memory from the body while others felt their discomfort was due to resistance to the Angelica's cleansing. Both may be happening. Erin, a student of plant spirit healing, developed physical symptoms several days after the Angelica ceremony. She gave this account at the time, outlining how she suspected it was linked to the Angelica working through her:

*For five of the last seven days I have had a fever accompanying a very tender head, spine, and sore neck. Sometimes I feel better and think I can get up and as soon as I am up for a little bit I feel exhausted and my symptoms flare. People have been concerned that there is something really wrong with me. I have thought maybe so too, but I also feel there is some serious Angelica work being done here. My dreams have been very vivid and I feel like they follow me into my daily reality (I am dreaming while awake walking around). The pain even increases in the night when I am sleeping and I wake up every night in the middle of the night at 2:00 or 3:00 a.m. wide awake for a while. I know that part of this is teaching me about nurturing myself and trusting in the Universe to take care of me. As painful as these past seven days have been and as concerned as people have been, I continue to have an overwhelming feeling that the plants are bringing me to my knees (in the last dismemberment I invited all my plant allies to work with Angelica and bring her in). Sometimes I think it is just me and I need to pull myself out of it but as soon as I start, life as usual pushes me down again. I am slowly surrendering and watching as the time passes and I am okay, maybe even better. It is still slightly scary though. I feel the plants caught me from slipping into the buzz of responsibilities of the material world . . . Oh, I also want to say that the pain and energy that shoots down reminds me of the light sabers from the pictures I took at Pam's place (see color plate 11, taken by Erin at the Angelica initiation).*

This account provides an example of the type of challenge that can occur as part of an initiation. The person is asked to surrender and let go of the illusion of control in order to move to a new level. You have to trust the process, surrender your ego, and wait it out in preparation for rebirth, growth, and expansion. In Erin's case, she created this dramatic scenario in order to take a massive leap forward in consciousness. Along with Angelica, she invited all her other plant allies to assist in the process, a powerful team! Always remember you can continue to ask for help from Spirit. In this instance Erin was calling on Angelica, Archangel Michael, and all of her other allies and helpers. Remember too, you can ask for gentleness and grace. A year later Erin revealed how much her life had changed, commenting, "Wow. Yes, that definitely was an initiation and afterward I let go of most of everything that came up from it. In this last year this cycle of initiation completed itself and I have been in the process of rebirthing myself. Angel Michael has stuck with me ever since."

## Types of Initiation

Typically, a plant initiation is most intense during the ceremony itself. Mary experienced the Angelica as "a tremendous surge of energy pulsing through my body" and said, "it was so powerful that I thought I wouldn't be able to contain it. Eventually, I felt my arms and legs fall away and I felt like I *was* Angelica with energy sparkling out of the top of my head. It was intense and wonderful." Similarly, Brenda shared:

> I felt the energy in the temple was so strong that I would disintegrate. I
> started feeling worse and worse; my body was aching, as were my teeth
> and gums and I was having trouble breathing. I lay down on the floor and
> went into a spontaneous dismemberment where I was completely flattened
> by a steamroller and when I closed my eyes, two thirds of my vision was
> deep blue and indigo, swirling around. The only dream I remember is that
> I had become a horse and was galloping free on the plains with a group of
> wild horses and really going for it. Now I have a huge sense of freedom and
> Light in my heart.

For Pam, who lives at Sweetwater Sanctuary, the intensity began two days in advance:

> I was presented with a particularly intense healing journey with Angelica as
> two days prior to the beginning of the initiation, I fell and broke my right
> wrist/arm. At first I was not sure I could participate as I was experiencing
> much pain, but I had a heart knowing that all was unfolding exactly as
> needed for my initiation. What I knew to be true was that I had been given
> a huge opportunity to work on very big issues in my life (loss of control,
> asking for help, patience, and being instead of doing, just to mention a few)
> while at the same time I was being initiated into becoming truly human,

*perceiving with my heart and taking up my rightful place in the vast web of Nature. After many other encounters with Angelica in the labyrinth, and through the practices of GreenBreath and dismemberment, the much grander winged presence began to be revealed. I have never had a particular affinity with angels, so don't relate to them as guides even though intellectually I have imagined that they exist. I also have balked at the association of Angelica with angels, thinking it was an old Christian throwback to times when the only help one could have was from an angel or a saint. When this magnanimous presence started hovering over the land, I asked Carole who or what this could be. She calmly replied, "Well that would be Archangel Michael, the patron of Angelica." I was stunned as my belief system reeled, slamming me into a reality I could not deny. The experience of such an omnipotent presence was overwhelming and yet brought about a magnificent state of grace. Now I know that Archangel Michael, with his sword of Light, is here at Sweetwater protecting and watching over this sanctuary and all who abide and visit here. What an amazing gift to be given by Angelica!*

I now end this chapter with words Angelica gave to Barbara:

> *I am snowy owl, Mother Angelica, Divine Mother.*
> *I beseech you to pray and in your daily prayers pray for*
>     *peace—peace in the world, peace in your heart, and*
>     *in every good work.*
> *Say your prayers daily and do not be afraid to die, for it*
>     *is in the dying that we are born again.*
> *Rise—rise up with the wings that have been given you,*
>     *each your own, for your own purpose.*
> *Not everyone is the eagle.*
> *Be mindful of the winged ones, they are here to remind*
>     *you that Spirit, love, Creator is ever-present.*
> *Take note. Make memory of the thoughts that come with*
>     *the birds, with the butterflies, and all creatures with*

*wings. Act swiftly and decisively with the message*
*that you receive. It is a gift to you from the Divine,*
*from Creator who loves you more than you know,*
*and from whom all good things come.*
*We are all one.*

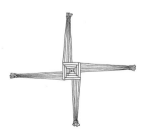

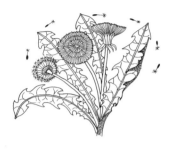

# 13

# Dandelion ☿ Spring Equinox
## Connecting Heaven and Earth

*D*andelion must be one of the world's most underappreciated plants! Denigrated as a weed and credited with causing bed-wetting merely by being picked, in truth Dandelion is an outstanding herbal medicine and a nutritious food, with an amazing storehouse of beneficial properties. Among the long list of medicinal actions, this valuable treasure is a powerful spring tonic and a highly effective cleanser for the liver and kidneys. Our liver is the major detoxifying organ in the body and in modern times this organ comes under enormous strain from the effects of stress, poor diet, and environmental toxins. Dandelion comes into its own as it cleanses and strengthens the human liver as well as the land itself. The plant sends its taproot into the earth, drawing up minerals while detoxifying the soil of heavy metals.

Described by Rudolf Steiner* as a "messenger from Heaven," Dandelion brings a wealth of gifts, both to earthly life and to our relationship with the Cosmos. This alchemical plant serves the interaction between Heaven and Earth, taking us out of ordinary time and into "no-time,"

---

*Rudolf Steiner (1861–1925) was an Austrian philosopher, social reformer, architect, and esotericist. He is the founder of biodynamics and his ideas formed the basis of anthroposophy.

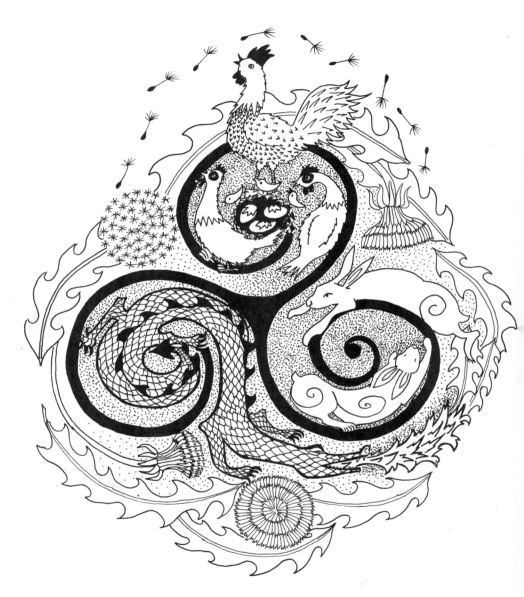

*The Spring Equinox is a time for celebrating new life, hope, and fertility.*

opening our awareness to symbol and dream. Ruled by expansive Jupiter and associated with the element of Air, the Dandelion seed head carries the ancient, archetypal pattern of the Flower of Life and under the right conditions it is reported that seeds may travel up to a hundred miles. The yellow disc of the flower brings an additional association with the sun and the astrological sign of Leo the lion, while the white sap and the silver globe of the seed head connect Dandelion with the moon. This is seen as a male plant, associated with the falcon, the opal, and the deities Hecate (Greek Goddess of the Crossroads and Magic, a protector of women) and Theseus (Greek hero god who defeated the Minotaur in the labyrinth).

Dandelions grow in human settlements; we are supposed to use them! In Steiner's opinion, just to have dandelions growing on a farm is beneficial. Dandelions are resilient, tenacious, and almost indestructible. Even a small piece of root left in the soil will regenerate. Rather than maligning them, we can rejoice and give thanks for their determination to be with us and we can make worthy use of the generous gifts they bring.

The brightly blooming Dandelion frequently bursts into color around the end of March, illuminating fields, roadsides, and garden lawns while offering us hope, vitality, and awakening. This messenger from Heaven has traditional associations with the Spring Equinox, holding a balance point between Heaven and Earth, and it is a perfect plant to diet with at this time. Dandelion represents the balance of instinct and intuition with the rational and logical. The coming together of heart and mind enables us to expand and move forward as sacred humans.

## SPRING EQUINOX
### Balance and Awakening

*Equinox* means "equal night." This occurs when the sun is positioned above the equator, causing day and night to be of equal length all over the world. The Spring Equinox falls around March 20–23 and is a time for celebrating new life, hope, and the activation of the fertility cycle. In Ireland and other temperate parts of the world, buds are bursting open, seeds are germinating, and eggs are hatching. It is a time to rebalance, break free, take risks, start new projects, and move forward. Our ancient ancestors are said to have honored the Spring Equinox in landscape-sized temples, such as at Mystery Hill in Salem, New Hampshire, where five standing stones and one recumbent stone are aligned with the Spring and Autumn Equinox sunrise. Researchers have concluded that this four-thousand-year-old megalithic site was erected either by Native Americans or by an unknown migrant population from Europe.

Eggs are a potent symbol of the Spring Equinox, representing rebirth, fertility, immortality and creation, and the potential promise of life. Easter, held on the first Sunday after the full moon after the Equinox, is intimately connected with this festival. The name Easter was a variant of the German/Saxon fertility goddess Ostara/Eostre (also the root of the words *estrus* and *estrogen*). Ostara was said to have mated with the solar God on the Spring Equinox and nine months later, around the Winter Solstice, gave birth to a child.

This is an ideal time to decorate eggs, either hard boiled or blown, with symbols of balance or pictures of what you wish to bring into the world. The eggs can be used to decorate your Equinox altar or they can be buried in Grandmother Earth who hears the cries and dreams of Her children. Gather with others around a sacred fire and pass around a hard-boiled egg, each focusing on all that you have been incubating over the winter and on what you desire to manifest. Offer this egg to the fire to activate and awaken your intentions. Sing and dance to call up the dragon energy that is rising at this time.

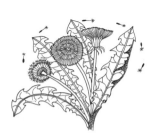

# DANDELION—MESSENGER FROM HEAVEN

*Taraxacum officinale*

**Plant family:** Compositae (Daisy Family).

**Other common names:** *Caisearbhan* (Irish); Lion's Tooth; Golden Suns; Burning Fire; Wet-the-bed; *Pis en lit* (French for Piss-the-bed); Shit-a-bed; Mess-a-bed; Wet-weed; Heart Fever Grass; Clocks and Watches; Blowball; Peasant's Clock; Fairy Clocks; Fortune-teller; Farmer's Clocks; Shepherd's Clocks; Time Flower; Tell-time; Twelve-o'clock; Witch Gowan; Devil's Milk Plant; Wild Endive.

**Description:** Dandelion is a hardy perennial that grows up to one foot high. It has a fleshy tap root, a hollow stem containing milky white latex, and deeply saw-toothed leaves that form a rosette at the stem base. Dandelions are fast growers, going from bud to seed in days, and they also live long lives. An individual plant can live for years and its root will delve deeper each year, going as far as fifteen feet down. The root clones when divided, and a one-inch piece of root can grow an entire new plant. Bright yellow flowers bloom from March to November, although in mild conditions the plants may continue to grow and bloom all year round. The flowers are followed by fluffy seed heads, the "Dandelion Clock," which is a ball of wind-borne seeds, each connected to a thin stalk and resembling a miniature parachute. The Dandelion is a prolific seed producer and a single plant can produce more than five thousand seeds a year. When released, seeds can be spread by the wind a long distance from their source.

**Habitat:** Dandelion is commonly found in gardens, pastures, lawns, meadows, waste ground, and on roadside verges. Dandelions can thrive in barren habitats and can push their way through gravel and cement.

**Distribution:** Said to have evolved about thirty million years ago in Eurasia (possibly originating near the Himalayas), the Dandelion now grows in temperate zones around the world and was widely spread by early European settlers. It was introduced to North America by early colonists in the seventeenth century.

**Species:** *Taraxacum* is a large genus of flowering plants with several hundred species worldwide. Even before the common Dandelion arrived with the Europeans, other species existed in North America up through Alaska, where there are Dandelion fossils dating back over a hundred thousand years. These are all safe medicinal plants and can be hard to tell apart. Despite being a common weed, Dandelion has a complex biology with many methods of reproduction. It can reproduce seed asexually, without pollen fertilization or any genetic involvement of male cells. It also can reproduce through insect pollination, self-pollination, and vegetative reproduction from roots.

**Parts used:** Leaves are best picked in spring. Roots can be harvested in autumn or for their juice in spring. Sap can be collected at any time and flowers appear in spring, summer, and autumn.

## Dandelion as a Spirit Medicine

As a Spirit Medicine, Dandelion has many faces. It always carries the gifts of the whole yet it may show itself in one particular guise, whatever is most fitting for the patient being treated. It may be that the root is prevalent: helping to release deeply held anger, guilt, resentment, and bitterness while bringing tenacity, determination, grounding, and inner stability. The leaves may come forward to cleanse emotions and balance our Water element, offering spiritual nourishment and renewal while enigmatically bringing both the courage of the warrior and sometimes a welcome release of tears. The sap reminds us who we really are, cutting through illusion and helping us dare to be different while the flowers bring rejuvenation, vitality, power, radiance, and the creative energy of the sun. The seed heads connect us with the stars, carrying messages from Heaven and opening us to spiritual guidance and blessings. We remember our soul's dream and are assisted in taking this out into the world. Both sap and seeds bring lunar energies, enhancing sensitivity and receptivity, helping the flow of our emotions, and teaching us about the law of cycles, including knowing when to move into a new phase.

All of these many qualities are present when working with the spirit of Dandelion. A mediator between Heaven and Earth, it offers expanded awareness and evolutionary change, bringing exactly what a person needs for his or her own transformation. It works simultaneously on the microscopic and the macroscopic levels: from our physical atoms and cells to our place in the expansiveness of the Universe outside of time and space. The Dandelion's metamorphosis from golden flower to an ethereal globe of seeds reflects this potent transformative power. Part of the transformation involves being in service and the Dandelion can be helpful in waking a person up to his or her soul's path of service in the world.

A tea of the leaves or a decoction of the root is taken to enhance psychic sensitivity and all parts of the plant are used in incenses, talismans, and amulets to invoke their respective properties. For lunar energies the seeds are best collected under the light of the full moon. Blessings can be sent to others by setting a firm intention and blowing upon a seed head.

## Dandelion as a Flower Essence

**Key words to describe this essence:**
Spiritual activation and expansion; grounding spirituality.

The following description refers to the Dandelion Crystal Skull essence, the making of which is shown in color plate 12. The photograph shows a bowl of Dandelion flowers being infused in the sun with a small crystal skull. This is a ceremonially energized skull that I have worked with for many years. Crystal skulls can have a variety of attributes including helping to raise our frequency and vibration. In the making of this particular essence it was clear that the Dandelions and the skull wanted to work together. The resulting essence is one that helps at times of massive expansion. An essence of both receiving and giving, it assists with grounding new patterns and strength, while simultaneously helping us to wake up and be in active service to others, able to give support with fearlessness and caring. Dandelion Crystal Skull essence activates our higher light wheels and enhances our connection with the stars while being firmly grounded on the Earth. It is restorative for crystals when used as a wash, bath, or spray.

## Dandelion in Folklore and History

Dandelion is one of our oldest medicinal herbs. Its use in medicine was recorded by Arab physician Avicenna in the tenth century and it has been consistently employed as a general curative, commonly given as a major remedy for the digestive system, especially the liver. In the Middle Ages it was used for eye conditions in Europe and in Germany it has been employed as a sedative since the sixteenth century. It has a history of esoteric connections and it is thought that the name *Dent-de-lion* (French for Lion's Tooth) may have heraldic or Kabbalistic origins. In England, before the First World War, Dandelion was grown as a commercial crop where the roasted, ground roots were sold for two shillings per pound to make into a drink. A similar beverage has a long tradition of use in Japan. At one time in Minorca, after other vegetation was destroyed by a plague of locusts, the islanders were forced to live on Dandelions.

In European folk tradition Dandelion has associations with time, and the seed heads are commonly known as Dandelion Clocks. Children around the world still blow on them to know the time. The number of puffs it takes to blow off all the seeds indicates the hour. Alternatively, to find out how long you have left to live, blow once on a dandelion seed head. The number of seeds remaining corresponds to the number of years you have left! The seed heads can also be blown on to find out if a lover is true. Say "He loves me, He loves me not" with alternate puffs and the final puff reveals the answer. Another custom is to make a wish and blow on the seed head. The wish will be granted if all the seeds are blown off with a single puff. Blowing on a Dandelion Clock can also send thoughts to a loved one. Visualize your message and blow in the loved one's direction. Burying Dandelions in the northwest of the garden is said to bring favorable winds and a method of calling to helpful spirits is to place a bowl of Dandelion root decoction beside the bed before going to sleep.

Dandelions are linked with the Spring Equinox as well as with Bealtaine (May Eve). Associated with Belenos (the Shining God) who was one of the most ancient and widely worshipped Celtic deities, they are one of the herbs of Belenos, or the *Belenountion,* yellow plants (including St. John's Wort) that are ritually gathered at midsummer in Brittany, France, and are said to form the body of the god. In England, Dandelion is linked with St. George, their patron saint who fought the dragon. It was customary to make Dandelion wine on St. George's Day, April 23, and St. George is considered a Christian version of a much earlier deity who overcame the dragon of winter and welcomed in the summer at Bealtaine. St. George is also an earthly representation of Archangel Michael, who, with his sword of truth, slays the dragon of our lower self in order to free the exalted dragon of our higher being (see chapter 12 for more on

Archangel Michael). In pagan traditions the deeply rooted Dandelion has also been associated with the underworld and linked with Samhain, when it is used to invoke Hecate, Greek Goddess of the Crossroads and Magic.

## *Dandelion in Contemporary Herbal Medicine*

Dandelion is a well-loved and frequently used plant of many herbalists, including myself. A famous liver tonic and diuretic, it cleanses the body at a cellular level and improves overall health with a versatility and gentle strength that make it highly valuable for a wide range of conditions.

Its actions are the sum of many different parts. A bitter principle is found in the whole herb and particularly in the root. Bitters are extremely beneficial to health and can be sadly lacking in today's diet. Their action starts with a bitter taste, stimulating bitter receptors in the mouth. This causes a reflex activation of the whole of the digestive tract including the liver. Dandelion root thereby enhances digestion, stimulating the liver, gallbladder, and pancreas while encouraging the secretion of digestive enzymes including stomach acids, bile, and pancreatic juices. This makes it helpful for nausea, indigestion, irritable bowel syndrome, and digestive bloating. Additional components in the plant stimulate liver, kidneys, and cell metabolism as a whole, making Dandelion one of the most far reaching of the healing herbs. Dandelion root has a particular affinity with the liver and gallbladder, being a highly effective remedy for a sluggish congested liver or any condition where there is a need to detoxify. It treats hepatitis, cirrhosis, and jaundice, relieves an inflamed gallbladder, and helps dissolve gall stones. Its extensive actions reduce high cholesterol especially when combined with artichoke. And its cooling and clearing properties can help lower high blood pressure when this is linked with congestion in the liver or poor blood circulation. By promoting the appetite, Dandelion assists during convalescence and is beneficial for the reduced appetite and lowered digestive functioning of advanced years. It stimulates the metabolism and can thereby help in a weight-loss program; it has a gentle laxative effect that relieves constipation and piles, benefits the spleen, and lowers raised blood sugar.

To make dandelion root decoction (or coffee as it is often called), the roots can be used fresh, dried, or roasted in a hot oven until dark brown. Roasting will give a nuttier flavor. It is best not to sweeten the drink since this reduces its bitter action. Taking the decoction daily over a number of weeks will have particularly beneficial effects.

By cleansing and stimulating the liver, Dandelion assists with tiredness, irritability, and headaches. It releases anger and resentment, often held in the liver, as well as relieving eye conditions such as itchy eyes associated with liver dysfunction. In depression, where anger is being turned in on oneself, Dandelion provides helpful liver cleansing and support and combines well with Lemon Balm or Skullcap. It is useful in a variety of gynecological conditions ranging from premenstrual syndrome and endometriosis to fertility and menopausal problems. By purifying the blood, Dandelion helps clear skin complaints such as eczema, acne, and psoriasis where it may be usefully combined with Burdock or Red Clover. It removes uric acid from the body, combining well with Celery seed or Nettles to treat gout. Dandelion benefits rheumatic conditions and is a wonderful treatment for degenerative joint diseases such as chronic arthritis. A powerful Dandelion cleanse can be undertaken in spring and autumn by juicing the whole plant (fresh root and leaves) to reduce stiffness, increase mobility, and help prevent further problems. Take up to a tablespoon two or three times daily for two weeks. Dandelion is antineoplastic and may be used as part of a natural cancer treatment, deeply cleansing the body and improving cell function.* It can also be used for viral infections, kidney stones, and to eliminate worms.

The whole plant, particularly its leaves, is rich in vitamins and minerals including beta-carotene, the precursor to vitamin A, vitamins B, C, E, and K, potassium, iron, and calcium. The leaves are a powerful diuretic, removing excess fluid from the body. They strengthen the urinary system, relieve fluid retention, and cleanse via the urinary tract. Nature has befitted the leaves perfectly for this task since they are remarkably high in potassium (nearly three hundred milligrams per one hundred grams).

---

*\*Antineoplastic* means "inhibiting or preventing the growth and spread of tumors or malignant cells."

This mineral is naturally eliminated from the body when we pass fluid and pharmaceutical diuretics require a potassium supplement to be taken at the same time. By taking Dandelion as a diuretic, any lost potassium is automatically replaced by the plant. The leaves are also used to treat bed-wetting in children and incontinence in older people. In Ireland, the fresh leaves (including their sap) are chewed to relieve severe coughs and asthma. The sap can be used directly on warts and applied daily for at least two weeks. It is also used to remove freckles, age spots, corns, unwanted hair growth, bee stings, and blisters. A simple way to conserve the sap is to pound the fresh stems with a mortar and pestle and mix this into a base cream or oil. The flowers make a useful infused oil for rubbing into tense muscles and stiff joints.

### Additional Uses of Dandelion

Dandelion leaves are a nutritious food. Delicious in salads, they can be added to soups and stews and cooked in innumerable ways. The buds can be boiled as a substitute for brussel sprouts and the flower heads are tasty when fried in butter. A delicate wine is produced from the flowers while roots, leaves, and flowers are all used for making beer. Consuming Dandelion blossom honey is a gentle way to receive the plant's benefits and an infusion of the flowers is used as a wash to remove freckles.

In Biodynamic agriculture, Dandelions are used in a compost preparation to enrich the soil. Dandelions are seen to impart their power to the compost, enlivening the soil and helping plants become more sensitive to their connection with cosmic forces. This facilitates plants to draw in what they need from a wide arena.

## PLANT DIETING WITH DANDELION

*After choosing to diet Dandelion, it is time to harvest the plants and prepare your elixir. Below you will find recipes for two Dandelion elixirs that I made at Derrynagittah. I have described the instructions that I received from Dandelion for making these two elixirs. When making your own elixir you will need to listen carefully to the plants and let them guide you. See chapter 4 for more complete information on harvesting plants and preparing the elixir.*

*In advance of your plant diet it is important to prepare yourself for several days with a period of physical and spiritual purification. At Derrynagittah we make specific cleansing and dietary recommendations for each diet. You will find the recommended preparations for the Dandelion diet below.*

## 🌿 MAKING THE DANDELION ELIXIR

You will notice that while most components in the elixir recipes below are expressed as parts of the whole, certain ingredients (notably vibrational essences) are listed with a specific quantity. In these cases, the amount is NOT proportional to the total amount of elixir and represents a quantity simply added to the whole. This is an intuitive, guided choice and the amount can remain the same, regardless of total quantity; that is, the same number of drops of essence can be added, whether to 20 oz. of elixir or 2 gallons.

*Elixir 1*

- 3 parts decoction of fresh Dandelion root and seeds (1 teaspoon of seeds was added five minutes before the end of the simmering)
- 1 part infusion of fresh Dandelion flowers and stems
- 2 parts infusion of fresh Dandelion leaves
- 2 drops Dandelion flower essence

**Amount of elixir taken at diet:** Six servings of 2 tablespoons and 2 teaspoons (50 ml) for each person

This elixir was prepared on the day of the Spring Equinox in 2012. I had risen early to be in the garden for the exact point of the Equinox (5:14 a.m.) in order to call in a new cycle for the garden. This is something I do every year and on this particular morning I was greeted by a multitude of stars, which revealed themselves in the dark sky as I entered the herb garden. Added to this was a symphony of bird song, a beautiful token of the awakening energies in the garden. Later that morning I explored the land, foraging for the Dandelions that had sprung up all around. While preparing the elixir, I received a lot of images and feelings about the connection between Heaven and Earth and in the middle of the ceremony to make the elixir I was interrupted by the uncommon arrival of a person in a van selling frozen food. Emblazoned on the outside of the van were the words "Heavenly Foods." An appropriate description for the Dandelion, I thought!

*Elixir 2*

- 3 parts decoction of both fresh and dried, roasted Dandelion root
- 2 parts infusion of fresh Dandelion leaves
- I part infusion of fresh Dandelion flower buds
- 10 drops Dandelion flower essence

**Amount of elixir taken at diet:** Seven servings of 2 tablespoons and 2 teaspoons (40 ml) for each person

For this elixir, the harvesting and making were done on the day after the Equinox and I had therefore done my calling in the day before. There was a great sense of new beginnings on the land and in the garden; the tangible feeling of starting a whole new chapter. On the sunlit morning of the Equinox I had walked the land and the eye-catching yellow discs of the Dandelion flowers could be easily spotted across the fields. They emanated sunshine and brightness. Today it was a different story. It was bitterly cold and, with the sun obscured by clouds, none of the flowers were open. Today I saw the moon side of their nature, and it struck me what an intriguing plant the Dandelion is with its mix of extrovert sunny energy and its more hidden lunar qualities. It seemed to me the perfect balance of light and dark, male and female, and yin and yang. Picking the Dandelions, I particularly noticed the star-like shape in the arrangement of their leaves and the abundance of their white milky sap, literally dripping down my fingers. I noticed, too, how they were the only plants shooting up through the paths we had carefully weeded last autumn. They're so commonplace we hardly notice them, and yet Dandelions are truly extraordinary!

## PREPARATION FOR THE DANDELION PLANT DIET

*General Preparations*

For three days prior to the diet take NO refined sugar, added salt, meat or dairy products, strong spices, coffee, alcohol, or fermented foods. Avoid oils apart from olive oil. Do not engage in sexual activity.

### Gentle Liver Cleanse

In addition to the general preparations, for the Dandelion diet we recommend a gentle liver cleanse for three days prior to the ceremony. Take 1 to 3 tablespoons of extra virgin olive oil with 3 times that amount of fresh lemon juice on rising each morning, followed by two glasses of the juice of a half lemon and hot water. Then either fast or wait one hour before having a simple breakfast of foods like oats, seeds, nuts, and/or fruit.

### Food during the Dandelion Diet

For those not fasting we recommend carrots, beets, and sunflower seeds.

### Suggested Drinks

We recommend Dandelion root or leaf tea, Ginger tea, fresh lemon, and hot or cold water.

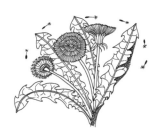

# DREAMING
# WITH DANDELION

*Through the alchemy of sacred ceremony and by surrendering to the plant, participants in a plant diet enter into an altered state in which they form close relationships with the plant that they are dieting and receive gifts that may be physical, emotional, mental, and spiritual. Many participants gain a completely new perspective on life. The relationship with the plant is deeply transformative, facilitating access to higher consciousness, guidance, and healing. In this section people who have dieted with Dandelion tell the stories of their personal transformations.*

## The Diverse Nature of the Dandelion

The multitalented Dandelion evoked a range of responses in our initiates, aptly reflecting its diverse nature. In the garden, Yukari observed the plant with awe and remarked on the beauty of its shiny, red-gold stem and how the leaves filled her with wonderment. Initially she felt scared by its "very strong will and so many seeds," but the fear was soon replaced by a "friendly feeling" and a sense of the Dandelion's "Light message." In Helen's words, "I just disappeared into the dream of the Dandelion with no push or pull. It was luscious and light and simply beautiful." For Katie, "It was a very visceral teaching: dropping into the deep yellow center and the stems; dancing in the wind; weaving the love of Grandmother Earth into my bones; weaving a new dance of celebration and gratitude for the manifestation of the dream; bringing in a deep communion of grace." Camilla described the plant's "physical strength and rootedness, teaching me the sense of being present in my body and to root down and sprout, trusting where I am and who I am, whatever the circumstances." Like many other initiates, Brenda shared how she was "moved by the gifts and blessings of the Dandelion and how underrated it is by the majority of us." Other typical characterizations included "hard-working," "persistent," "tenacious," "playful," "loving," and "happy to be shared." Its energy was generally encountered as male, with descriptions varying from "a loving man with dark hair and a beard," "a lovely old man like my grandfather or the scarecrow in the Wizard of Oz," to "a man who dances a lot with an upturned head, a thin body, and a dandelion skirt."

## Deep Cleansing and Transformation: Knowing We Are Enough

The Dandelion cleansed us on all levels: physical, emotional, mental, and spiritual. For Katie, the plant

*released the binding of the mind and gave me an experience of pure love, dropping me into the freedom your elixir brings, merging with Dandelion, and going beyond the fragmented despair and isolation; going beyond judgment. There was a great freeing of stuck patterns in my body. I felt the*

*light coming through and freedom coming back into form, like when I am*
*in a warm ocean and really trusting that I belong and that I am enough.*

The sense of being enough was echoed by Brenda who recalled, "During the night I was waking up at times and observing old beliefs and patterns and seeing different circumstances and that my previous views were mistaken. I saw the words *I am enough* and was urged to remember this. I felt the Dandelion very companionable, a strong and reliable friend." The letting go of judgment was reiterated by Helen:

> *When I first took the Dandelion I could feel it rushing through my whole being, telling me to drop the judgmental side of the mind and come back into the heart. After the blessing outside I was anxious as to whether I would be able to come back to my heart. I felt dreamy and wanted to close my eyes and when I did a song came to me. It was about love and how every time you feel down or discouraged, think of the vibrant yellow of the Dandelion. There was permission to just be and allow things to be as they were. It was a relief that I did not have to talk and could just be expansive in nature. The message when taking it again was to "think big and leave the fear and allow myself to dream."*

Mary Teresa described an intense experience where Dandelion explained that while she could not change past events, she could change her feelings about them and thereby transform them. She recalled:

> *As soon as I sat down after taking the Dandelion it focused on my head and I could feel it moving around. Later on I felt really exhausted and when I met the Dandelion in the journey, I felt a great pain where it was moving around and something burst in my head. I fell asleep and woke up with a splitting headache, which I had for hours. The Dandelion spoke to me of obstacles in life and that we may not be able to get rid of them, but we can grow around them. There was a big realization that what has happened in the past cannot be banished with recapitulation since those things will always be a part of us, but we can bend and twist around them and still come through.*

*Later on I had a really powerful experience where the Dandelion helped me clear obstacles in the form of mistaken beliefs and then gave me a wonderful gift. I first met a huge monster in human form. He was really solid and kept saying, "You are not good enough." I started cutting through him with my sword and eventually he was just a mass on the ground, moving and oozing and burning with vile liquids bubbling and seeping out of him, trying to get away until eventually he was just dry ash on the ground. I felt I was heading for a beautiful place and then I saw another creature on my path and he was very wiry and hard to pin down, scrawny. He said, "You still can't do it." I couldn't catch him and eventually I spun a thread around him and then I sliced him with my sword and then I burned him. Again there were pieces of him trying to crawl away. I thought I was finished and I met another creature like Gollum and he was the hardest of all, really cunning.\* He jumped behind a tree. I kept wondering who and what he was. I grabbed him by the head and stuck the sword through his chest and he sizzled and as he did so the form went out of him and then I burned him. He represented self-doubt.*

*An ancestor from the Sidhe led me to a grove of trees and in the center was a golden shining Light, the essence of the Dandelion.† I felt it washing through my body and out into my auric field. It penetrated the essence of my soul and it was the most perfect pleasure. I became formless; then I was on my knees in the form of a wolf. Sometimes my head was human and my body wolf. It kept changing. Sometimes I was stroking the wolf even though I was the wolf. I felt great love and peace in knowing who I was. I was running through the land and there were other wolves and I felt at home, contented, and at peace.*

## Supporting Our Soul's Dream

Many accounts reflected how Dandelion helped initiates to know and walk the dream of their soul. Helen shared how she had specifically asked for guidance with her dream:

---

\*Gollum is a fictional character from Tolkein's *The Hobbit* and *The Lord of the Rings*.
†Sidhe is another name for the Tuatha de Danaan, or People of the Goddess Danu, an ancient race of Ireland.

*While I was drinking the elixir, I had asked, "What is my soul's dream in connection with the plant world?" I have a big connection with Mount Shasta [in California] and during the weekend I was taken there and to County Clare [in Ireland] and to Hornby Island [in Canada]. I was walking through the trees and it felt like Heaven on Earth. A stag came and I changed into a dove and it was the sacred marriage of the two. This has given me a lot of information to work with.*

For Danu, a budding actress, Dandelion encouraged her to persevere with her dream. She shared:

*Last Christmas I lost hope in my dream. I lost faith in everything, wondering if maybe I wasn't good enough. I felt confused but I decided to try for one more year. This year I have felt more energy and more opportunities are coming my way. I am in four plays and I have had a promotion. I am trying to believe in myself. Dandelion grows anywhere and everywhere, nothing can stop it. It's telling me, "You cannot give up or stop. You have to keep pushing yourself." The Dandelion is not suffocating other plants. It's not hurting anyone. It has real strength to push through and transform. It tells me that now is the time to keep going and to move forward with my dream.*

Another initiate, Emer, painfully expressed, "my dream was killed." She explained that she had spent years "compensating," going on to say:

*This morning something came through and I started to understand. I have never expected to be deserving of good things. I felt unworthy; unloved; not truly cherished. I've accepted that and therefore I've accepted that there is something wrong with me. It's an innate aspect. This understanding has been a revelation and at this moment I am calling on the Dandelion for guidance, for dreams. Right now I feel much more grounded.*

Earlier that morning Emer had encountered a physical stag while out walking (many wild deer live around this land) and the animal stood gazing at and connecting with her for many minutes. This sacred meeting reminded Emer of her own power and majesty, bringing a message from the otherworld of her grace, strength, and intrinsic value. Interestingly for us, the stag has connected repeatedly with the Dandelion diets, being frequently mentioned by initiates. Stag is a regal creature with enormous dignity, power, and integrity; the King of the Forest.

## Receiving Insights and Navigating Obstacles

Dandelion gave insights into our current behavior patterns as well as advice about navigating the obstacles in our lives. For Amanda, information was revealed through an experience from a past lifetime:

> *Dandelion removes blocks, eases tension, makes one more manifest in the body, and makes known the reasons why one is resistant to embodiment, including offering visions into previous life trauma. In my own experience, I saw a lifetime where I felt powerless. I revisited the pure shock of certain traumas from that life and I saw where these energies still hook me.*

For Suzy, Dandelion brought healing for her heart, a message of self-acceptance, offering significant insights into how best to proceed in her life. She gave this account:

> *The Dandelion took me on a journey to the heart and the fire that is the heart; the heart fire. I felt I was blowing on a horn, calling to someone or something. A huge stag on top of a mountain came. I was asked to let go and my body started to shake. I heard the words "Shake it sister. Move your body." I began to weep deeply. This is the wound of the heart. It began so early in life. It needs mothering and it needs the white sap of mother's milk that is the Dandelion. It needs the power and protection of stag and to know that it can be healed, but it takes the courage of lion, Fire to burn through it all, Water to cleanse it, wind to blow through it. I got great solace from realizing that my body will heal. I felt deeply loved by this little plant. In the past I have been blown away by sadness and despair. This weekend helped the healing of the wound of the heart and showed me how I can choose to mother and nourish myself and how to*

*put boundaries around all my negative beliefs. I felt deep happiness. The Dandelion said, "It's ok to feel angry. Own your emotions. Happiness is a balance of emotions." It reminded me of Rumi's poem,* Guesthouse, *where he talks about welcoming all the guests, even those who may trash your house.\* Dandelion says this to me: to accept all parts of myself.*

Barbara received insights around seeds, noting, "the seed contains the hologram of the Whole. I can see the importance of planting new seeds, being freed of old patterns and beliefs, and just getting on with what you want to do. I have a new consciousness of Dandelion as an ally and I love that." Camilla was inspired to do her "shaking" practice with the Dandelion, referring to "shaking medicine," a spiritual practice from India that involves shaking one's body. She told how the Dandelion made her aware of her core issues and helped her not to be afraid.

## Interconnectedness and Spiritual Awareness

In common with other plant initiations, there was a theme of interconnectedness. Suzy realized she was "already connected with the Dandelion" and said, "I have the realization of the interconnectedness of Dandelion, how we're all separate but interconnected." Observing the plants, Yukari felt "their message was to live together." This was reiterated by Camilla, who shared the message, "We can live in close proximity to nature and to others." Katie reported, "I was dreaming with the Dandelion and it was a very visceral teaching of the understanding of community and the web that has always been holding Grandmother Earth."

Many participants commented on their awareness of spiritual presence. Yukari said, "I could feel the spirits were with us in the temple. When I closed my eyes I felt the presence of other beings next to me and when I opened my eyes there was nobody there," and Danu shared, "I felt two people come and lay down beside me." Yukari recounted a dream:

---

\*Rumi is a thirteenth-century Persian poet and Sufi mystic.

*This building [the temple] is on top of a mountain and we are looking at another mountain opposite. The view is like from an airplane; it's really beautiful. Then someone says, "There's a fire, the mountain is burning," and we see that smoke is coming out of the other mountain. It's like a volcano about to erupt. Many angry-looking bears are escaping from that mountain. They are very upset and they are coming toward us. I was very frightened. It was a very emotional dream.*

Yukari, who is Japanese, explained that in Japan, bears are held sacred and can signify God. On reflection, she felt that the mountaintops represented a high spiritual dimension and that the dream illustrated how Spirit was coming to her and this made her feel afraid. She was being offered a chance of embracing Spirit or God. She felt it showed an underlying fear of surrendering to Spirit and of taking the next step and gaining deeper intimacy with the spiritual realm. These kinds of fears can easily come up at plant initiations. My suggestion was to ask Dandelion for help and to work with the bear on the inner planes to develop a harmonious relationship.

## Symbols, Cellular Change, and Working with Time

Dandelion had a particular propensity to bring symbols to the initiates. Maeve, an artist, shared, "a symbol came that represents the Dandelion bringing Heaven to Earth and I was told to incorporate this in my current art project." Brenda received a symbol that she was inspired to express in a planting design in her garden. Several people received images of body cells and referred to cellular purification or reorganization taking place. Camilla commented, "The Dandelion restores order to cell structures within the body." Katie described the plant as "purifying the DNA of disconnections, projections that have kept me from the mystery, the magic of my essence." Suzy recounted, "I keep getting the image of the seed and its long, very delicate, wispy protrusion. It looks like a cell body. Its delicacy reminds me of a nerve cell with its axon and the dendrite that makes connections from nerves to muscle.

I can feel in my body that the seed sends out messages every time it goes out."

Time took on a new meaning with Dandelion. Many people not only lost track of time, they were generally disorientated, and some reported major changes in their usual senses of place, direction, sight, hearing, taste, and smell. Amanda felt that Dandelion was able to affect time by harmonizing the timelines and helping to bring past, present, and future into greater accord. She gave this account:

> *Even though many view Dandelion as a common weed, it is powerfully connected to the timelines. Its whirling, radial pattern itself indicates a harmonic. Working with Dandelion can help bring the timelines themselves into greater harmonic accord (versus the lines looking chaotic or tangled), which again is a clearing of blocks within the greater organization of the Universe. As the timelines are brought into greater accord, blocks will be cleared in the past as well, and all parts of the self will come into greater harmony with each other. Dandelion also helps with daily navigation, helping one to see his/her way around obstacles when they are presented. Dandelion showed me not only blocks in my own body, but where I cut myself off from love. It also helps remove blocks to growth or metamorphosis.*

### Altered States and Visionary Experiences

For some, the Dandelion initiation resulted in a major alteration of consciousness. This is my own account:

> *The ceremony went from easy to hard in a split second. I felt like Dandelion completely took me over. Before the drumming session I was feeling really sick and later on I went into an altered state. I had drunk water and it reminded me of being in Peru at a plant diet where we took a preparatory plant beforehand and drank lots of water in order to purge our systems and to make us more receptive. It made me wonder if Dandelion could also be beneficial if used like that before dieting with another plant. By the end of the drumming I was feeling so ill that all I could do was stop and*

*lie down. As soon as I closed my eyes vivid pictures started coming. First of all I was inside the fluid of a cell looking at this big round hairy object that I knew was a virus. It was like being inside a 3-D electron microscope picture of a cell. Then I saw a woman sitting holding a sick baby on her lap. She said, "The antibiotics aren't working" and I had the sense that she meant globally they weren't working, like major antibiotic resistance had developed in the world. The message was that Dandelion could help, that it was both antiviral and antibacterial. I was bringing up a lot of mucus and I felt the dandelion was cleansing my physical body, clearing out the residual effects of a flu I had several weeks earlier. These are not typical properties I associate with Dandelion. At one point I saw Garlic cloves, which may have meant that I need to take Garlic, although it would also be a useful herb to explore as part of an anti-infective combination with Dandelion.*

*I lost track of time, sounds were greatly amplified, and I was alternating between being boiling hot and shivering with cold. I also saw galloping black stallions with shiny coats where I could feel their softness, and there were other visions that I can't remember. It was a beautifully clear night and I felt a powerful calling from the stars, Mars and Jupiter in particular. During the night the moon was so bright, shining in the window, a perfect half moon. Usually I love being in the moonlight but this time it made me feel even worse and I had to turn away. It was different than any moonlight I had seen before. The moon kept turning into a Dandelion head and showering me with Dandelion seeds and sap at the same time. This entire experience was more akin to the kind of experience one might encounter with a psychoactive plant like Ayahausca and clearly demonstrated the amazing power and potency of Dandelion, a so-called weed. I felt Dandelion had so much to share and it was absolutely determined to get its message across.*

After this experience, I am left with the complete certainty that we are only just beginning to realize the potential of Dandelion. It grows quietly all around us and is carrying powerful medicine that can help our consciousness to evolve and that may yet assist our physical survival in unknown ways. I am definitely inspired to explore its possibilities as an antiviral/antibacterial agent. As Katie put it, "It's so wonderful to come to a place within myself of honoring and appreciation of Dandelion's medicine. Indeed, it's time to dream deeply with her simple and constant manifestation of hope and beauty, remembering the part of humanity that can grow wherever it wants to."

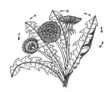

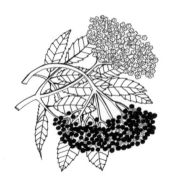

# *14*
# Remembering Who We Are
## *Manifesting Heaven on Earth*

*A very good vision is needed for life, and the man who has it must
follow it—as the eagle seeks the deepest blue of the sky.*

CRAZY HORSE, LAKOTA LEADER
AND VISIONARY (CA. 1840–1877)

From the Beauty Way teachings comes a lovely expression called "growing corn." Considering that corn is a staple food for millions of the world's population, it is clearly an extremely valuable plant and the term *growing corn* refers to the planting and cultivation of precious seeds. These seeds are our own gifts—our potential—the inspired ideas, dreams, teachings, and skills that we are supposed to plant, nourish, and grow. Like any responsible gardener or farmer, we want to care for our seeds and do the best we can to encourage them to thrive. In this tradition it is understood that the gifts we receive in life are meant to be put to use, our innate talents and capabilities are intended to be cultivated so they can flourish and contribute to the well-being of our world. Regardless of our individual gifts, all are equally valuable. By nurturing the seeds we are given, we can truly realize our potential and nourish

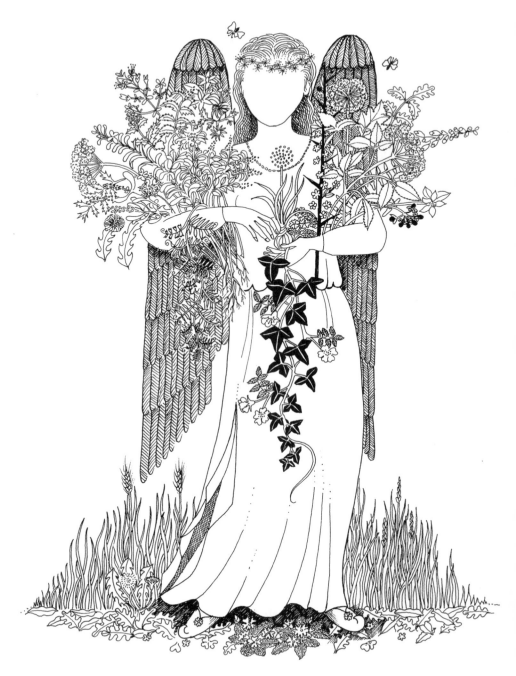

*Plant angel*

both ourselves and the world. In the same vein, the actions we take, the thoughts we choose to entertain, and everything in life can be viewed as "growing corn" or otherwise; beneficial to life or not. Therefore, for any action, the question arises: "Does this grow corn?" "How does the step I am taking contribute to the well-being of the world?"

With these thoughts in mind, I studied the longer-term effects of the plant diets, looking at the impact they have had on people's lives and exploring the lasting consequences. For me, these plant initiations have been life changing and I wanted to hear how other initiates had fared. Some of the effects are immediate while others unfold over time. I was interested to know what changes had occurred and how these affected people's lives in a tangible way.

I am happy to report that this research has overwhelmingly confirmed for me that the plant initiations are genuinely helping people to transform their lives for the better and are subsequently benefitting their wider communities. Some of the longer term effects have been touched upon in previous chapters, such as in chapter 11, "St. John's Wort," where Fernanda describes how she subsequently transformed her eating habits, and in chapter 12, "Angelica," where April outlines several concrete developments in her healing practice that arose from the plant diet she attended. Tracking the consequences of the initiations has revealed a long list of lasting beneficial effects, too lengthy to include in its totality, but I will do my best to summarize the key areas.

One point to mention is the beneficial effect of the simple pleasure that people frequently feel from spending "quality time" in ceremony with a plant. In April's words, "I was nearly drunk with happiness at the opportunity to spend three days in ceremony with plants, spirit beings, and humans." Brenda shared:

*I realized how much I love both being with plants and being in ceremony. At one of the plant diets I thought to myself, "These things give me so much pleasure. Why don't I make them more of a priority?" The plants have shown me that I don't need to suffer and instead I am supposed to follow what makes me happy. Since this revelation, I resolved to do just that and consequently I have felt an enormous sense of peace and fulfillment. It has significantly improved my life.*

Pat described how she felt "privileged to spend dedicated time with a sacred plant being; held in a safe, sacred space and sharing this with other humans." She went on to say, "Being in community is important for me and from doing the plant initiations I have since been guided to participate in other community groups."

Each plant dieted is experienced as having its own specific temperament, qualities, and emphasis, while at the same time several common themes have arisen from all the plant diets. This is true for the initiations described in this book as well as those with different plants we have dieted.

## TRANSFORMING OUR RELATIONSHIP WITH PLANTS AND NATURE

*We are on the brink of a revolution that will reunite humans with nature.*
DAVID ATTENBOROUGH, ENGLISH BROADCASTER
AND NATURALIST (1926–)

One of the most widely reported effects of these ceremonies is the profound transformation of our relationship with plants and Nature. The plant initiations deepen our relationship with Nature. The form this takes is specific to each individual. Anna said she has become "more aware and remembers that plants are also alive," while Nicola reported, "I have been on a journey for some time to connect more deeply with plants and Nature. The diet really helped me to ground this in an Irish context." Naira shared, "My whole approach has changed," explaining that

*the plant initiations have helped me in finding the sacredness within the plants. Helping me to relate to them in a more personal and respectful way, understanding their spirituality more rather than just their physical appearance. At the same time, I now understand how many ways we can relate to plants with absolutely all of our senses. We can enjoy smelling them, eating them, hugging them, touching them, or just sitting and enjoying their presence, being open to receiving what they can bring.*

Henrique described how his connection with all of Nature has deepened:

*My relationship with Nature has changed; not only with plants, but with animals too. I don't feel like eating meat as I did before. Now, if I do, I want to know where the meat comes from and how the animal is being treated. I can say the same for plants and vegetables. How are they being cultivated? Now I feel my connection with all beings on a deeper level.*

Linda, a veteran at our plant diets, has formed a deep and committed relationship with plants. She said, "My relationship with flowers, plants, herbs, and trees is deeper and stronger. I feel blessed, delighted, and full of wonder and so much joy. They are so beautiful and so generous. I pray for the elementals and devas of all the plant world that they may be strengthened and blessed, protected and honored."

Pat, who moved to a new home some months earlier, commented, "the diets have changed my relationship with my own land. I have been able to anchor myself here much more than ever before and I can feel its sacredness." Amanda described how she would never look at plants in the same way again:

*During the plant diets, we learn that being connected to these beings is not to look out or at them but to be in the dream with them. We don't just deduce their healing properties or shift our abilities to perceive, we hear the plants speak. Through our bodies, we become their transcribers. I didn't realize until working with plant diets that each plant is a book. The* messages of each plant are vast and complex, dynamic and irreplaceable. I will never look at the plant world in the same way after participating in this work. I now have a burgeoning sense of the wild specificity of each of these creatures and of how they each hold an integral part of the planetary web. I have been touched by them.

Sal, an advanced student of plant spirit healing, revealed that since the plant initiation, "my psychic abilities have been blown wide open and I am receiving an abundance of spirit guidance." She added:

One of my intentions going into our Angelica initiation was to deepen my connection with the green beings. The shift I experienced has been profound. My felt sense of awareness has become clearer and stronger, which blesses me with much more insight into the glorious plant world. I have experienced the plants reach out to me more and more. I hear their messages more clearly. It is so wonderful!

For Anais, an herbalist, the Angelica plant initiation helped her to develop a deeper relationship with Angelica as an herbal medicine. She said:

I have a much better idea of how to use Angelica and it works wonders when I recommend it for health troubles. For example, I gave it to my sister who at twenty-eight had almost never had a normal period. It was always scanty, spaced apart by months, and generally only ever happened when she lived with other women with a strong hormonal lead. Taking the pill did not even provoke periods. So I gave her a mix including Angelica and four weeks later she had a normal period. She continued to have normal periods until I changed her mix because she had acne and wanted it controlled. I added liver plants and forgot to keep Angelica in. She was only menstruating every two months with the new mix, and not very abundantly. As soon as I put the Angelica back in, it returned back to normal.

For Terri, the plant initiation has put her on a new path. She shared, "I can definitely say that my relationship with the plant world has opened up. I am more observant of plants at seasonal times; I notice things I didn't see before. I am working more closely with plants, growing herbs, trees, and flowers as well as my own vegetables. This is now my chosen path in life."

Erica, who has attended several plant diets, had this to say:

*Goodness, where to start about life changes since the plant diets! That could probably be the subject of a book on my own part! Here is what comes to me now: life has changed immensely. I now see plants and trees in an altogether different way. I am filled with respect for them. I have come into relationship with them. I have deep love and gratitude for them. I continue to be awed and graced by the gifts they bring. I have a deep desire and need to spend time in nature every day, often in the woods, or along quiet country lanes, or by the sea. Often, I feel called to stop in a particular location to spend time with a plant or tree and I frequently take the opportunity to tune my light wheels then and there.*

*Probably all of the plants I dieted with have become allies for me. Oak reminds me of my inner strength and helps me to be strong. Dandelion has helped enormously over the last year in detoxing and cleansing my digestive system. I have been taking the herb in its dried root form. Nettle has been a great tonic for me. I was in my element making a tincture of young leaves and shoots last spring. Elder has helped notably with ancestral healing and feels like a very dear old friend. How I loved harvesting the bountiful berries last autumn and making medicinal syrup and jelly with them. Blackthorn has reminded me profoundly of who I am and has awakened great healing in, and through, me. Elecampane recently accompanied me in clearing very difficult and entrenched ancestral issues pertaining to the lungs and grief. Hawthorn, too, is a strong ally and has come vividly in my dreaming. Like Blackthorn, Hawthorn reminds me of who I am. Nowadays, I meditate and/or journey with my plant allies every day. I am noticing in particular how they are helping me change long-standing chronic patterns and move toward more robust health and well-being. It feels like I am being entirely renewed from the inside out! And I sense that my work in the future will be very different from what I did in the past.*

## WORKING WITH PLANT ALLIES

*Gratitude is not only the greatest of virtues but the parent of all others.*
CICERO, ROMAN PHILOSOPHER, POLITICIAN,
LAWYER, AND ORATOR (106–43 BCE)

A natural consequence of these initiations is that we become more aware of plants as allies. Echoing Erica's experience, following a plant diet it is common to find that the plant in question will offer itself as a longer term ally. Pat described how Oak and Dog Rose have stayed with her as plant allies:

*Oak brings me great strength, stability, and generosity of spirit. I feel its spirit in my heart and I feel I am more tolerant and compassionate. Dog Rose comes with so much beauty. At the time of the initiation, she taught me about being in community. But now she is there as a lightness and a feeling of dancing my life, not plodding along, which I am inclined to do. I feel her in my third light wheel.*

April said, "Since the Angelica initiation, I have often felt the presence of the Angelica spirit. Sometimes the feeling comes unbidden; perhaps a scent brings her close, or instead it's a glimpse of white flowers in a distant field. More usually, it's because I call on her, as I do when I feel the need for angelic protection for myself or my loved ones." Carmel, who has worked with plants for some time, revealed:

*I now have a different relationship to the plants I've worked and journeyed with. I feel a bond with them. I am aware that we are connected on an energetic level and they are there for me when I open to them. Also, when I ask for guidance and allow it to come, it does so in the most unexpected ways. I've received clear guidance about living from the heart, turning toward the Light, and igniting the fires within.*

Estelle, who attended a Blackthorn diet, recounted that she is now much more conscious of the power of plants to protect, heal, and guide her. She continued, "Since the diet I can feel and smell plants in Nature and sometimes in my dreams too. Blackthorn is now an ally and teacher for me. She shows me the different parts of my personality and teaches me about parts of myself that are blocked." Naira is also aware of receiving guidance from plant allies. She commented, "Now when looking for guidance or answers, I feel the plants are allies who remind me of my true essence, backing me up so I feel more rooted to make decisions." Anna described how Blackthorn made practical suggestions: "She wants me to use her wood in any way I like. After the plant diet I made some Blackthorn runes and since then I have gotten deeper into working with runes." Blackthorn has also become an ally for Grainne who shared, "Happily, there are several Blackthorns in our garden. I have recently made a seat under one tree, which I use when I need to connect to my core self. Sitting there helps me to think clearly from a rooted place. The Blackthorn nurtures my emerging crone and helps me to feel my own strengths."

## DEEP HEALING AND SELF-DISCOVERY

*Your soul longs to draw you into love for yourself. When you enter your soul's affection, the torment in your life ceases.*
JOHN O'DONOGHUE, IRISH POET, PHILOSOPHER,
AND CATHOLIC SCHOLAR (1956–2008)

In chapter 10, "Elder," Jane described how her long-standing back pain cleared during a plant diet and then stayed away afterward. Some people report the immediate and lasting improvement of physical health issues while some, like Erica above, describe a more gradual improvement of chronic health problems. In these cases, there is an improvement initiated at the plant diet that then continues over time. Added to this, there are countless reports of long-term benefits to all aspects of health. Henrique said, "My health has improved in a general way since the diet: mental, physical, emotional, and spiritual." Pat reported feeling much less anxious, more trusting, and more joyful in her life in general. Maura told of a "heaviness of spirit" that has now lifted while Carmel described having inner shifts that are "subtle but definite—a general movement within, like my being is slowly tilting into alignment at all levels (physical, emotional, spiritual)."

Lindsey offered this account:

*The Angelica plant diet has been profound in helping move the grief and guilt that I carried with me from learning the history of my ancestors. The initiation has given me many, many tools of learning and healing that I am reminded of and drawn to on a daily basis, and which help me to come back into my whole self. Angelica really helped heal the mental and emotional picture of my own body and self in ways that have provided essential foundational shifts. These new images of self come to me when I am playing out old tapes or finding myself triggered by a situation that resembles the past. I have these images of myself as whole; not lacking, victimized, hurt, or incomplete in any way. I still have self-defeating thoughts and feelings, but I am now a person who, when I experience them, has tools: new tapes and mantras to play instead of negative mind chatter.*

Mary Teresa, a regular participant at the plant initiations, gives a summary of her experiences:

*The plant diets have taken me on a journey of deep healing and self-discovery. The plants, always generous in their giving, brought me to places I had never been before. In times of confusion, they showed me a way through. In times of desperation, they offered me refuge. Through visions and dreams they brought answers to my questions and relief to my inner longings. They showed me how to cut through the obstacles I had created in my life. They guided me through the layers of grief and loss and brought me to a new understanding of life and death. We are all part of the natural ebb and flow of life. They guided me on journeys deep within, helping me to find that still point and bringing me to a deeper knowing of my true self. They brought me to other realms and other levels of consciousness. Through their vibration, they taught me how to connect deeply with the Earth and to trust in her refuge, to bury my roots deep within her and to stay grounded and connected. They taught me to turn my face to the sun and to receive its blessings and to give thanks, how to be at one with all in Nature. They have shown me how to look at the world from a different perspective. They have healed wounds deep within me and they have brought healing to those that are close to me. I have been blessed by their generosity.*

## EXPANDING CONSCIOUSNESS AND COMING HOME TO OURSELVES

*I must be willing to give up what I am in order to become what I will be.*
ALBERT EINSTEIN, GERMAN THEORETICAL
PHYSICIST (1879–1955)

The self-discovery described by Mary Teresa is echoed by many others. As Naira said, "The plants remind me of my true essence." She went on to explain that now, if she feels scattered or fragmented, she is able to call on the plants to bring her back to herself. Henrique reported a similar dynamic, in his case associated with an enhanced awareness of spirit guidance. He said:

*I've begun to receive guidance more clearly, especially when my mind is very noisy. I can clearly hear the voices of my guides and guardians pulling me back to my natural state, giving me some advice or encouraging words. I always felt their presence and their help, but now it is becoming more and more clear. I think one of the reasons for that is because my conscious awareness has increased.*

April explained how the plant initiation helped to reunite her with an underdeveloped part of herself:

*The first most powerful and recurring theme of the plant-dieting experience was reunion with what I'll call "the priestess" part of my being—the one who wholeheartedly participates in sacred ritual. Since the initiation, I have felt not only driven but also empowered to foster in my life the impulse to create ceremony with people and nature beings. I recently offered my first workshop, Communing with Tree Spirits. It is almost as if I'm a novice priestess being trained by the plants and my plant spirit healing teachers. From time to time I feel compelled to kneel in the presence of a tree or plant and I get a tangible sensation of hands being placed on my head in benediction.*

Carmel described how she now finds it easier to go with the flow of life saying, "There's been a shift in my consciousness and I trust the flow more. One of the changes is that I can let go more easily and just accept the way things come and go, without fighting." Brenda, another veteran of our plant initiations, described how the ceremonies have helped her to grow and evolve:

*The plant diets have helped me to grow up. There's been immense healing and I have released a lot of grief. I think this was possible only because I felt so much love from the plants and it enabled me to trust and let go. Also, in a loving way, the plants have been showing me my shadow aspects, highlighting all the unhelpful, destructive, and unpleasant behavior that I engage in. They made me realize that these patterns weren't working, helping me to own and accept my shadow, to integrate all of that, and to embrace who I am. Not that I don't sometimes slip into old patterns, but it's very different now. It's like observing an old part of myself and gently reminding myself of what's real. Now I can connect with a more evolved part of me who gives encouragement, reassurance, and comfort to the old frightened part, explaining the meaning of what she's going through and helping her to deal with it. It's like a wise and loving parent, which is also how I experience the plants.*

## INTERCONNECTEDNESS: BEING INITIATED AS A SACRED HUMAN

*To love somebody is a commitment that says, "I will not forget who you are," and "I will not abandon you," and "Together, we will remember what is real."*

ROBERT HOLDEN,
ENGLISH PSYCHOLOGIST,
AUTHOR, AND BROADCASTER (1965–)

The sense of our interconnectedness has been mentioned in many of the previous chapters, such as in chapter 8, "Oak," where Ian describes receiving "the realization of connectedness, wholeness, and Oneness with everything and everyone." Here, Camilla recalls her experience of being part of the Web of Life:

*The effects of such a weekend are subtle and gentle, but very real. Reality is not that of a made-up film world of TV and video, but of a very fine living web in which we and Nature are integral parts, living side by side. We need to start living sooner rather than later within this dynamic relationship of self, Nature, and the human world. The weekend I spent with Elder has been a gentle birthing into this dynamic.*

Henrique, who said he now felt a deeper connection with all beings, went on to describe how he perceives the changes within himself to be affecting others close to him. He explained, "What is interesting is that people around me have started to change some of their negative habits and I associate this with the Light that the St. John's Wort carries, and that I now carry, in my heart. I really feel my heart is beating stronger for life now and it's affecting my surroundings in a positive way." He continued, "I'm definitely very different, in a positive way, and I can now feel and perceive the subtle connections of all that manifests in my life. I can only be very grateful for who I am, for being alive, and for the gifts that life gave me."

Maura shared that the plant initiations have given her "a new view of reality":

> Now I see plants as allies who help us and I see Spirit in all things. I've realized that we're all interconnected parts of a larger web where each being is unique and valuable. It has made me feel much better about myself. I know that help is always available and that I am never alone. I would say I am more confident and self-assured, less ego-driven. I like the focus on gratitude that we have at the plant diets. It has made me much more aware of the importance and benefits of giving thanks for everything in life. On a practical level, the diets have changed my whole approach to gardening. I am now much more sensitive and aware of the invisible realm.

In the next account, Dalton outlines how a Primrose initiation helped him to grow as a person:

> When I did my first plant diet I already had an introduction into plant spirits and journeying; not much, but enough to feel confident that doing a plant diet would be a comfortable next step. What happened over that weekend has helped me to grow as a person and to feel more a part of this world and connected with others as a result. Experiencing the plant diet has definitely put a better perspective on life, on what is important, and on how much we as human beings are so much a part of the web of life, more than I ever thought possible. It may be obvious to some that we are part

*of everything, but without that experience it would not have appeared so obvious to me as it does now. My plant diet was with Primrose. I prepared for the diet not expecting anything in particular or having preconceived notions, just with a willingness to experience and explore something new and to basically have a fun weekend. Since the diet I have certainly grown in many ways. I have a deeper love and appreciation for all things living, and in particular plants. Their generosity and understanding is something I can only describe as like having a patient teacher helping me deal with difficult situations and problems that I either face within myself or in life, situations I find myself in. I've learned to love myself more and appreciate my own beauty; a task I never thought possible before, as I thought that self-loathing and the inability to improve were normal. I have had a good relationship with plants for quite some time, but now my perception of the plant world is certainly different. When I think of plants now I think of them as friends, others who we share this Earth with. I'm now aware of the possibilities of what we can all share and learn from each other. I believe my experience has helped me to become more confident, more assertive, kinder, more understanding and open, and without fear of humiliation. I'm now continually trying to better myself. That said, it certainly hasn't been the easiest journey as I've been made to look at myself and ask difficult questions. Often the way I am led in order to help myself seems to be full of difficulties and challenges, but I believe it is through facing these challenges that I've become a better person.*

Brenda reflected that through the plant diets, she is learning how she can be of better service in the world:

*The plants have shown me that by fully being themselves, they nourish and activate the self in others. It's a kind of teaching by transmission. I've realized that the same applies to humans and the more I am fully myself, the better I can serve the planet. Just like a flower whose mission is simply to bloom, my mission is simply to be myself. All I have to do is love and accept myself and know that I am enough. That way I give myself permission to enjoy my life and to enjoy the expression of my dream. The plant diets are helping me to get closer to expressing the fullness of who I am and I've realized that I can make a difference in the world simply by being me. It's so simple and so liberating. I am very grateful to the plants. They are amazing.*

For myself, I echo Brenda's words. I know the plant diets are helping me to be in service, both to my own personal dream and to the world. I continue to be taken ever deeper into the plant world, delighting in our relationships and astonished by the generous gifts offered. I have received enormous healing, support, and guidance. I have been inspired and nurtured, restored and uplifted, both through my own experiences and through the privilege of sharing the experiences of others. At times the initiations have been massively challenging, but always this has been part of an extensive healing process for which I am forever grateful. Completely outstanding is the profound and enduring unconditional love that the plants carry. To experience such love can truly change lives. I notice I am becoming kinder to myself and others. The plant diets are helping me to remember who I am and that love is all there is. More and more, I can radiate that reality out in the world. As a healer and teacher, I am consistently better able to embody the wisdom of the plants and thereby assist my clients and students, as well as the collective. I can hear the plants more clearly and I can do a better job of bringing their messages to others. They are clarifying my vision of how to be in service and helping me to identify practical steps to make this happen. Moreover, I can see that these ceremonies are benefitting the wider world—the benefits are reaching out into the community and helping to bring positive change. They are indeed "growing corn."

## REMEMBERING THAT LOVE IS ALL THERE IS

*There are only two ways to live your life. One is as though nothing is a miracle. The other is as if everything is.*

ALBERT EINSTEIN

Many people are either openly worried or secretly uneasy about the state of our planet, but most of us feel powerless to make a difference. Some of the news is so heart-wrenchingly painful that people simply close their minds to what's happening. Amid a bewildering array of advice, we simply don't know what to do for the best, with the result that we often do nothing. At the same time, we instinctively know that Nature holds the key to our survival, that of course we are a part of Nature and cannot be separated from it. Reconnecting with plants and Nature is a critical and crucial step for humanity. By forging that connection, the plant diets are massively valuable, helping us build a respectful, loving relationship with the plant world. Plants are some of the most ancient beings on this planet and are intimately connected with humans. We even share the same DNA coding system. Plants provide us with food, medicine, shelter, warmth, and oxygen to breathe. They give us life itself and we cannot live without them. Restoring a healthy relationship between plants and humans is of urgent importance, and following the methods described in this book is one way to make that happen.

Plant consciousness wants to be recognized. It guides us through inspiration and dreams, so-called coincidences, and chance encounters. At this significant time on the planet, plants are coming forward with exactly what we need, and it is time for us to pay attention. Furthermore, connecting with plants in this way can help to make our lives so much more fulfilling. Plants can help us to develop into mature human beings and remember how to be in service. Plant initiations not only make us feel good, bringing guidance and healing, they also expand our consciousness and take us to a whole new level of being. Here, we can interact with the vast, creative knowledge of all that is and we can be of service in restoring the intricate web of life that has been disrupted by human activity. We can truly learn to walk this Earth as sacred humans, living in harmony with all the worlds of Grandmother Earth and serving the collective for the greater good.

I have had the immense good fortune of being immersed in the plant world for most of my life. In this book I have attempted to share with you some of the many gifts offered by the plants. In my daily life I continue to be astonished, amazed, and inspired by all that the plants bring. I hope that I have done them justice as their spokesperson and that you too have been inspired. I trust that I have been able to show the benefits of the plant initiations and to demonstrate the pure love that is carried by plants and how this can help us to evolve as sacred humans. I encourage you to embrace what is written and to find the time to practice some of the skills that resonate most strongly with you. Applying the knowledge in this book can bring rich benefits. The plants can help us to transform our lives and our world. Most important of all, plants show us unconditional love. They remind us of the sacred law that "love is all there is" and offer us the personal experience of being loved without judgment or condition. Love is the way forward for us as a species. By surrendering to love and merging with that which is greater, human consciousness can expand in ways that we have hardly dared to imagine. It is time to remember that we are made of love. This is who we are and this is our destiny. It is my heartfelt prayer that this book will help to heal the relationship between humans and Nature and help all of us to awaken and remember who we are.

*Sacred Child of the Cosmos, Divine and Sacred Human,*
*Come now and step through this Gateway to the greater*
    *reality.*
*Open your heart with gratitude,*
*Surrender to the unconditional love of the plants,*
*Journey deep into the vastness of Self.*
*Join in ecstatic communion with the plant world,*
*Dance with joy in the abundant flow of consciousness,*
*Let the plants reflect your exquisite Beauty within.*
*You are Divine in your own right.*
*Bask in the brilliance of your Divine Soul,*
*Shine your radiant Light as a guide to others.*
*Sacred Star-Seed of the awakening Dream,*
*Remember who you are!*

*Access the wisdom of your Soul,*
*Be the embodiment of Heaven on Earth,*
*Be the embodiment of Love.*

*May this book grow corn in a way of beauty, heart, grace, peace,*
    *and freedom.*

### BLESSED BE

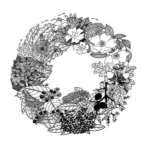

# APPENDIX I

# Deities Mentioned in This Book

**Áine:** Irish Goddess of Love, Fertility, Summer, Wealth, and Sovereignty.

**Airmid:** Tuatha Dé Danaan herbalist and healer, daughter of Dian Cécht.

**Aphrodite:** Greek Goddess of Love, Beauty, Pleasure, and Procreation. Equivalent to the Roman Goddess Venus.

**Bacchus:** Roman God of Wine, Winemaking, and Ecstasy. Equivalent to the Greek god Dionysus.

**Balder:** Germanic God of Nature, Summer, and Light. Son of Odin and Freya.

**Banbha:** Tuatha Dé Danaan sister of Éiru and Fódla. Goddess of Sovereignty.

**Belenos:** Celtic god (the Shining God) worshipped from Italy to Britain, associated with fire and pastoralism. His symbols are the horse and the wheel.

**Blodeuwedd:** Welsh Goddess of Flowers, magically created to be the wife of Llew.

**Brigid (Bride, Brid):** Daughter of the Dagda, keeper of the sacred flame and holy wells. Irish Goddess of Poetry, Smith Craft, and Healing.

**Christ:** Commonly treated as synonymous with Jesus of Nazareth, the name translates to "the Anointed One."

**Cupid:** Roman God of Desire, Erotic Love, Attraction, and Affection. Equivalent to the Greek god Eros.

**Daghdha (Dagda):** Irish Father God of the Tuatha Dé Danaan (the people of the Goddess Danu—mythical, divine inhabitants of prehistoric Ireland). Son of Danu, He is a master of magic and keeper of the sacred cauldron of abundance.

**Danu:** Irish Mother Goddess of the Tuatha Dé Danaan (the people of the Goddess Danu—mythical, divine inhabitants of prehistoric Ireland).

**Demeter:** Greek Goddess of Corn, Grain, and the Harvest; Earth, Agriculture, and Fertility.

**Donar:** Germanic equivalent of the Norse god Thor.

**Éiru:** Tuatha Dé Danaan Goddess of Sovereignty who serves as an eponym for Ireland. She forms a triple goddess with sisters Banbha and Fódla.

**Eostre:** *See* Ostara.

**Eros:** Greek equivalent of Cupid.

**Fódla:** Tuatha Dé Danaan sister of Éiru and Banbha, Goddess of Sovereignty.

**Freya (Freyja):** Norse Goddess of Love, Sexuality, Beauty, Fertility, Gold, War, and Death.

**Hathor:** Egyptian Goddess of Love, Beauty, Joy, Motherhood, Sky, Foreign Lands, Mining, Music, and Fertility. Often depicted as a cow goddess with horns, linked with Venus/Aphrodite.

**Hecate:** Greek Goddess of the Crossroads, Entranceways, Magic, Witchcraft, the Night, and the Moon. Associated with plant medicine and childbirth, a protector of women and the oppressed.

**Herne:** Commonly considered equivalent to Cernunnos, the Celtic Horned God. In English folklore Herne the Hunter is a ghost who rides in Windsor Forest with antlers on his head.

**Hymen:** Greek God of Marriage Ceremonies, inspiring feasts and song.

**Isis:** Egyptian Goddess of Motherhood, Magic, and Fertility, and Children. A patroness of Nature and protector of the dead.

**Jupiter (Jove):** Roman King of the Gods. A sky god of thunder and lightning, equivalent to the Greek Zeus.

**Kwan Yin (Guanyin):** East Asian Goddess of Compassion, she is a bodhisattva, an enlightened being who stays in human form because of her compassion for the suffering of other beings.

**Lugh (Lug):** Tuatha Dé Danaan hero and Sun God, Lugh of the Long Arm, renowned for his many skills and gifts as a craftsman. A harvest god and God of Blacksmiths and Artisans.

**Maeve (Medbh):** Celtic Warrior Goddess, faery queen, and Goddess of Sovereignty. Associated with magic, intoxication, protection, leadership, justice, fertility, and power.

**Morgan le Fay (Morgane):** Celtic Queen of the Fairies, Goddess of Battle, Fertility, and Sexuality. A sorceress, shape shifter, and healer with knowledge of herbal medicine.

**Morrigan:** Powerful Celtic phantom queen and Warrior Goddess of Battle, Strife, and Sovereignty. Shape shifter, death bringer, and Goddess of Fertility.

**Ostara (Eostre):** Germanic Goddess of the Radiant Dawn. Associated with the month of April.

**Shekinah:** Wisdom Goddess of the Kabbalah, the Old Testament, and Merkavah mysticism.

**Theseus:** Greek hero god who defeated the minotaur in the labyrinth.

**Thor:** Norse God of Thunder, Lightning, Storms, Oak Trees, Strength, the Protection of Mankind, Healing, and Fertility.

**Thunor:** An alternative Anglo-Saxon name for Thor.

**Venus:** Roman Goddess of Love, Beauty, Sex, Fertility, and Prosperity; a vegetation goddess and patroness of gardens and vineyards. Daughter of Jupiter. Equated with the Greek goddess Aphrodite.

**Zeus:** Greek God of the Sky and Thunder, presiding deity of the Universe, ruler of Heaven and Earth, personification of the laws of Nature, father of gods and men, and lord of state life.

# Summary Steps for Performing a Ceremonial Plant Diet

Below is a quick summary of the steps taken in a ceremonial plant diet. Detailed instructions can be found in chapter 4.

1. Set your intention and decide which plant to diet.
2. Harvest the plant and prepare the component parts of the elixir. If your elixir is simply one part, for instance a single infusion or decoction, then this stage will include step 4 below.
3. Prepare yourself by following a cleansing regime for at least three days prior to the initiation.
4. Do a final ceremonial mixing of the component parts, adding prayers of blessing and intention.
5. Prepare and purify your ceremonial space, asking permission from Spirit, setting up your altar, and gathering whatever you will need for the duration of the plant diet. For instance you will probably want a sleeping bag and cushions, a notepad and pen, a CD player or similar technology for playing music, and perhaps drinking water, art materials, a drum, or other instruments.
6. Prepare and purify yourself, ensuring that you will not be disturbed during your diet.
7. Center yourself, focus your intent, and if you have a pack of divination cards, intuitively select a card that can help guide you in this ceremony.
8. Now with clear intent, call to whatever guardians and spirit

helpers you choose to invoke. This is the start of your ceremony.

9.  Pour some elixir and offer it as a gift to Grandmother Earth.

10. Now pour some for yourself (or for the group if you are in one), surrender to the plant, and take your first drink. From this point onward, you will be dreaming with the plant, whether awake or asleep, and periodically drinking the elixir (you choose how much and how often). You can use the audio files available at audio .innertraditions.com/saplin to travel with the plant; you can journey with other sounds or with silence; you can spend time with the plant outside in nature. You may like to breathe with the plant, to sing, dance, or express the plant through writing, drawing, or other creative means. The choice is yours and the plants will guide you. Record your experiences and review these at the end. If you are in a group, share your experiences on the last day.

11. When it is time to close the ceremony, thank and release all the beings who have helped you.

12. Finish with a celebratory feast.

13. Afterward keep a seventy-two-hour discipline or integration period (see chapter 4 for details).

# APPENDIX 3

# Plants Associated with Each Fire Festival

Below is a list of plants associated with each Fire Festival. This is intended to give you ideas for your own seasonal plant diets. It is by no means exhaustive or rigid. As always, the key is to be guided by the plants and to allow yourself to be inspired!

## BEALTAINE

Almond (*Amygdalus communis*)
Apple (*Malus* spp.)
Ash (*Fraxinus excelsior F. americana*)
Betony (*Stachys betonica*)
Birch (*Betula alba*)
Broom (*Sarothamnus scoparius*)
Cinquefoil (*Potentilla reptans P. canadensis*)
Clover (*Trifolium* spp.)
Dandelion (*Taraxacum officinale*)
Daisy (*Bellis perennis*)
Deadly Nightshade* (*Atropa belladonna*)

Elder (*Sambucus* spp.)
Hawthorn (*Crataegus* spp.)
Honeysuckle, Woodbine (*Lonicera caprifolium*)
Hop (*Humulus lupulus*)
Horse Chestnut (*Aesculus hippocastanum*)
Ivy* (*Hedera halix*)
Lady's Mantle (*Alchemilla vulgaris*)
Marigold (*Calendula officinalis*)
Meadowsweet (*Filipendula ulmaria*)
Mugwort (*Artemisia vulgaris*)
Oak (*Quercus* spp.)
Primrose (*Primula vulgaris*)
Rose (*Rosa* spp.)

---

*Deadly Nightshade is poisonous and should not be taken internally unless under the supervision of a medical herbalist.

*Overdosage of Ivy can be toxic. Seek guidance from an herbalist for internal use.

Rowan (*Sorbus aucuparia*)
Sweet Cicely (*Myrrhis odorata*)
Willow (*Salix* spp.)
Woodruff (*Galium odoratum*)
Wood Sorrel (*Oxalis acetosella*)
Yarrow (*Achillea millefolium*)

## SUMMER SOLSTICE

Angelica (*Angelica archangelica*)
Ash (*Fraxinus excelsior F. americana*)
Chamomile (*Chamomilla recutita; Chamaemelum nobile*)
Chickweed (*Stellaria media*)
Chicory (*Cichorium intybus*)
Cinquefoil (*Potentilla reptans; P. canadensis*)
Daisy (*Bellis perennis*)
Elder (*Sambucus* spp.)
Elecampane (*Inula helenium*)
Fennel (*Foeniculum vulgare*)
Feverfew (*Tanacetum parthenium*)
Figwort (*Scrophularia nodosa*)
Hemp* (*Cannabis sativa*)
Honeysuckle, Woodbine (*Lonicera caprifolium*)
Lavender (*Lavandula* spp.)
Male Fern† (*Dryopteris filix-mas*)
Marigold (*Calendula officinalis*)
Meadowsweet (*Filipendula ulmaria*)

---
*Seek guidance from an herbalist for internal use of Hemp.
†Seek guidance from an herbalist for internal use of Male Fern.

Mint (*Mentha* spp.)
Mistletoe* (*Viscum album*)
Mugwort (*Artemisia vulgaris*)
Pine (*Pinus* spp.)
Rose (*Rosa* spp.)
Rosemary (*Rosemarinus officinalis*)
Skullcap (*Scutellaria lateriflora*)
St. John's Wort (*Hypericum* spp.)
Sunflower (*Helianthus annus*)
Sweet Cicely (*Myrrhis odorata*)
Thyme (*Thymus* spp.)
Vervain (*Verbena officinalis*)
Yarrow (*Achillea millefolium*)

---
*Overdosage of Mistletoe can be toxic. Seek guidance from an herbalist for internal use.

## LUGHNASADH

Apple (*Malus* spp.)
Alder (*Alnus glutinosa*)
Basil (*Ocimum basilicum*)
Berries of all kinds
Borage (*Borago*)
Chicory (*Cichorium intybus*)
Corn (*Zea mays*)
Daisy (*Bellis perennis*)
Fennel (*Foeniculum vulgare*)
Fenugreek (*Trigonella foenum-graecum*)
Gorse (*Ulex eurpaeus*)
Heather (*Calluna vulgaris*)
Hollyhock (*Althaea rosea*)
Honeysuckle, Woodbine (*Lonicera caprifolium*)

Ivy* (*Hedera halix*)

Lady's Mantle (*Alchemilla vulgaris*)

Marshmallow (*Althaea officinalis*)

Mistletoe† (*Viscum album*)

Mugwort (*Artemisia vulgaris*)

Nasturtium (*Tropaeolum majus; T. minor*)

Oak (*Quercus* spp.)

Oat (*Avena sativa*)

Sunflower (*Helianthus annus*)

Thyme (*Thymus* spp.)

Valerian (*Valeriana officinalis*)

Yarrow (*Achillea millefolium*)

---

*Overdosage of Ivy can be toxic. Seek guidance from an herbalist for internal use.
†Overdosage of Mistletoe can be toxic. Seek guidance from an herbalist for internal use.

## AUTUMN EQUINOX

Alder (*Alnus glutinosa*)

Angelica (*Angelica archangelica*)

Apple (*Malus* spp.)

Ash (*Fraxinus excelsior; F. americana*)

Basil (*Ocimum basilicum*)

Berries of all kinds

Blackberry (*Rubus villosus*)

Blackthorn (*Prunus spinosa*)

Blessed Thistle (*Cnicus benedictus*)

Corn (*Zea mays*)

Daisy (*Bellis perennis*)

Elder (*Sambucus* spp.)

Ferns (various)

Hazel (*Corylus avellana*)

Hawthorn (*Crataegus* spp.)

Honeysuckle, Woodbine (*Lonicera caprifolium*)

Ivy* (*Hedera halix*)

Marigold (*Calendula officinalis*)

Milk Thistle (*Carduus marianus*)

Myrrh (*Commiphora mol-mol*)

Oak (*Quercus* spp.)

Passionflower (*Passiflora incarnata*)

Rose (*Rosa* spp.)

Sage (*Salvia officinalis*)

Walnut (*Juglans regia*)

---

*Overdosage of Ivy can be toxic. Seek guidance from an herbalist for internal use.

## SAMHAIN

Alder (*Alnus glutinosa*)

Apple (*Malus* spp.)

Aspen (*Populus tremula*)

Bay Laurel (*Laurus nobilis*)

Blackthorn (*Prunus spinosa*)

Broom (*Sarothamnus scoparius*)

Catmint, Catnip (*Nepeta cataria*)

Corn (*Zea mays*)

Elder (*Sambucus* spp.)

Fumitory (*Fumaria officinalis*)

Hazel (*Corylus avellana*)

Hop (*Humulus lupulus*)

Ivy* (*Hedera halix*)

Juniper† (*Juniperus communis*)

---

*Overdosage of Ivy can be toxic. Seek guidance from an herbalist for internal use.
†Avoid internal use of Juniper if you have weak kidneys.

Lavender (*Lavandula* spp.)

Mugwort (*Artemisia vulgaris*)

Mullein (*Verbascum thapsus*)

Nettle (*Urtica dioica*)

Nightshades* (plants of the
Solanaceae Family), such as
Bittersweet, Deadly
Nightshade, Henbane,
Datura, Tobacco

Oak (*Quercus* spp.)

Pumpkin (*Cucurbita* spp.)

Rosemary (*Rosemarinus*)

Rowan (*Sorbus aucuparia*)

Rue† (*Ruta graveolens*)

Sage (*Salvia officinalis*)

Skullcap (*Scutellaria lateriflora*)

Valerian (*Valeriana officinalis*)

Vervain (*Verbena officinalis*)

Wild Garlic (*Allium ursinum*)

Wormwood (*Artemisia absinthe*)

Yellow Cedar, Tree of Life (*Thuja occidentalis*)

---

*These plants of the Nightshade Family can be deadly poisonous and should not be taken internally unless under the supervision of a medical herbalist.
†Internal use of Rue can be toxic and the plant can irritate sensitive skin. Seek guidance from an herbalist.

Bay Laurel (*Laurus nobilis*)

Birch (*Betula alba*)

Blackthorn (*Prunus spinosa*)

Blessed Thistle (*Cnicus benedictus*)

Chamomile (*Chamomilla recutita; Chamaemelum nobile*)

Cinnamon (*Cinnamomum zeylanicum*)

Cloves (*Eugenia caryophyllus*)

Elder (*Sambucus* spp.)

Fir, Silver (*Abies alba*)

Frankincense (*Boswellia thurifera*)

Hazel (*Corylus avellana*)

Holly* (*Ilex aquifolium*)

Ivy† (*Hedera halix*)

Juniper‡ (*Juniperus communis*)

Marigold (*Calendula officinalis*)

Mistletoe§ (*Viscum album*)

Oak (*Quercus* spp.)

Pine (*Pinus* spp.)

St. John's Wort (*Hypericum* spp.)

---

*Holly berries are strongly purgative. Seek guidance from an herbalist for internal use.
†Overdosage of Ivy can be toxic. Seek guidance from an herbalist for internal use.
‡Avoid internal use of Juniper if you have weak kidneys.
§Overdosage of Mistletoe can be toxic. Seek guidance from an herbalist for internal use.

## WINTER SOLSTICE

Apple (*Malus* spp.)

Ash (*Fraxinus excelsior; F. americana*)

Aspen (*Populus tremula*)

Bayberry (*Myrica cerifera*)

## BRIGID'S DAY/IMBOLC

Alder (*Alnus glutinosa*)

Alfalfa (*Medicago sativa*)

Angelica (*Angelica archangelica*)

Basil (*Ocimum basilicum*)

Bay Laurel (*Laurus nobilis*)

Birch (*Betula alba*)

Blackberry (*Rubus villosus*)

Celandine, Greater* (*Chelidonium majus*)

Celandine, Pilewort (*Ranunculus ficaria*)

Chickweed (*Stellaria media*)

Coltsfoot (*Tussilago farfara*)

Heather (*Calluna vulgaris*)

Iris, Blue Flag (*Iris versicolor*)

Rowan (*Sorbus aucuparia*)

Tansy (*Tanacetum vulgare*)

Violet, Sweet (*Viola odorata*)

Wild Garlic (*Allium ursinum*)

Willow (*Salix* spp.)

---

*Overdosage of Greater Celandine can be toxic. Seek guidance from an herbalist for internal use.

## SPRING EQUINOX

Alder (*Alnus glutinosa*)

Apple (*Malus* spp.)

Ash (*Fraxinus excelsior; F. americana*)

Birch (*Betula alba*)

Bistort (*Polygonum bistorta*)

Blackthorn (*Prunus spinosa*)

Broom (*Sarothamnus scoparius*)

Celandine, Greater* (*Chelidonium majus*)

Celandine, Pilewort (*Ranunculus ficaria*)

Chickweed (*Stellaria media*)

Cinquefoil (*Potentilla reptans; P. canadensis*)

Cleavers (*Galium aperine*)

Coltsfoot (*Tussilago farfara*)

Daisy (*Bellis perennis*)

Dandelion (*Taraxacum officinale*)

Elder (*Sambucus* spp.)

Gorse (*Ulex eurpaeus*)

Ground Ivy (*Glechoma hederacea*)

Honeysuckle, Woodbine (*Lonicera caprifolium*)

Iris, Blue Flag (*Iris versicolor*)

Jasmine* (*Jasminum officinale*)

Lovage (*Levisticum officinalis*)

Marigold (*Calendula officinalis*)

Mugwort (*Artemisia vulgaris*)

Nettle (*Urtica dioica*)

Oak (*Quercus* spp.)

Pine (*Pinus* spp.)

Rose (*Rosa* spp.)

Tansy (*Tanacetum vulgare*)

Violet (*Viola odorata*)

Walnut (*Juglans regia*)

Willow (*Salix* spp.)

---

*Jasmine berries are poisonous and should not be taken internally.

---

*Overdosage of Greater Celandine can be toxic. Seek guidance from an herbalist for internal use.

# How to Use the
# Plant Initiation Audio Tracks

The audio tracks that accompany this book (available at audio.innertradi tions.com/saplin) are designed to be used at a plant-diet ceremony. Prepare for the ceremony as outlined in the book and play the audio tracks once you have started the ceremony. Be sure that you are in a comfortable place, either sitting or lying down, and have a cup of your elixir ready to drink at the start. The first track is a guided journey that brings the plant into your wheels of light or energy centers. More information on these centers is given on page 287. The narrative on the audio tracks will guide you through the wheels of light and the different sounds will help you explore each of these gateways with your plant. The second track is an instrumental, mystical journey designed for dreaming with the plant (awake or asleep). The third track is a guided journey taking you to meet your plant in nature. This is a drum journey with narration at the start and end. As before, you need to be in a comfortable position for this journey. The fourth track is a recording of a St. John's Wort Plant (Tutsan) singing through a plant biofeedback machine and is suitable for dreaming with any plant. You can go through all of the recordings in one session or you can listen to the individual tracks in your own timing, interspersed with other activities.

1. Bringing a plant into the Wheels of Light (34:46)
2. Mystical Journey (14:52)

3. Journey to meet a plant in Nature (19:53)
4. Plant Song (5:16)

## THE WHEELS OF LIGHT

Light wheels are the energy centers located within and around the body. These vortices of energy have different names in different spiritual traditions but are commonly referred to as *chakras* from the Sanskrit word meaning "wheel of light." Various traditions accord differing qualities and positions to these subtle energy centers. Here, I am describing the first ten wheels of light as presented in the teachings of medicine woman Arwyn DreamWalker and Navaho Grandfather Tom Wilson. Each of the light wheels are equally valid and important as they correspond to different aspects of life and act as gateways to other realms of consciousness. Their nature and positioning can be briefly described as follows:

Light wheel 1: Base of spine; color red; element of Fire
Light wheel 2: Pelvic cradle; color orange; element of Earth
Light wheel 3: Navel; color golden yellow; element of Water
Light wheel 4: Heart; color emerald green; element of Air
Light wheel 5: Throat; color electric blue; element of Ether
Light wheel 6: Third eye; color indigo; ancestors/self-concept
Light wheel 7: Crown; color violet; the dream
Light wheel 8: Whole body; color black velvet; cycles and patterns
Light wheel 9: Auric field; rainbow colored; design of energy
Light wheel 10: Eighteen to twenty-four inches above head; color diamond-white light; all mind/one mind

## CREDITS FOR PLANT INITIATION AUDIO TRACKS

Written and performed by Rory Guyett, Josh Guyett, Carole Guyett, Henrique Pederneiras, and Tutsan. Recorded, mixed, and mastered by Josh Guyett and Rory Guyett. Copyright © 2014 by Rory Guyett, Josh Guyett, and Carole Guyett.

# Resources

### *Aura Soma*
A form of soul therapy using color, plants, and minerals.

www.aura-soma.net

### *GreenBreath*
A method of deepening one's relationship with plants developed by Pam Montgomery, of Sweetwater Sanctuary, Vermont.

www.partnereartheducationcenter.com

email greenpam@vermontel.net

### *Vibrational Essences and Sprays*
A vast selection is available worldwide. My own range of Derrynagittah essences includes essences and sprays for all the plants featured in this book and can be purchased through my website. There is also a wide selection of additional essences and room and aura sprays.

www.derrynagittah.ie

# Bibliography

This list contains sources that I have referred to, as well as suggestions for further reading.

Barker, Julian. *The Medicinal Flora of Britain and Northwestern Europe*. West Wickham, U.K.: Winter Press, 2001.

Barnard, Julian. *Bach Flower Remedies: Form & Function*. Hereford, U.K.: Flower Remedy Programme, 2002.

Barnard, Julian, and Martine Barnard. *The Healing Herbs of Edward Bach: An Illustrated Guide to the Flower Remedies*. Bath, U.K.: Ashgrove Press, 1995.

Bartram, Thomas. *Encyclopedia of Herbal Medicine*. Dorset, U.K.: Grace Publishers, 1995.

Beryl, Paul. *The Master Book of Herbalism*. Custer, Wash.: Emer Publishing Co, 1984.

Bruton-Seal, Julie, and Matthew Seal, *Hedgerow Medicine*. Ludlow, U.K.: Merlin Unwin Books, 2008.

Carding, Emily. *Faery Craft: Weaving Connections with the Enchanted Realm*. Woodbury, Minn.: Llewellyn, 2012.

Carr-Gomm, Philip. *DruidCraft: The Magic of Wicca and Druidry*. Lewes, U.K.: Oak Tree Press, 2013.

Carr-Gomm, Philip, and Stephanie Carr-Gomm. *The Druid Plant Oracle*. London: Connections, 2007.

Culpeper, Nicholas. *Culpeper's Complete Herbal and English Physician*. London: Harvey Sales, 1981.

Cunningham, Scott. *Cunningham's Encyclopedia of Magical Herbs*. Woodbury, Minn.: Llewellyn, 1985.

De Cleene, Marcel, and Marie-Claire Lejeune. *Compendium of Symbolic and Ritual Plants in Europe*. Ghent, Belgium: Man & Culture Publishers, 2003.

Findhorn Foundation. *The Findhorn Garden*. Dyke, U.K.: Findhorn Press, 1975.

Fitter, R., A. Fitter, and M. Blamey. *Wild Flowers of Britain and Northern Europe*. London: Collins, 1985.

Goldstein, M., G. Simonetti, and M. Watschinger. *Complete Guide to Trees and Their Identification*. London: Little, Brown, 1990.

Grieve, Maud. *A Modern Herbal*. London: Penguin, 1980.

Hoffman, David. *The Holistic Herbal: A Herbal Celebrating the Wholeness of Life*. Dyke, U.K.: Findhorn Press, 1983.

Hopman, Ellen Evert. *A Druid's Herbal of Sacred Earth Year*. Rochester, Vt.: Destiny Books, 1995.

Houghman, Paul. *The Atlas of Mind, Body, and Spirit*. London: Gaia Books, 2006.

Ingerman, Sandra. *Medicine for the Earth: How to Transform Personal and Environmental Toxins*. New York: Three Rivers Press, 2000.

Kaminski, Patricia. *Flowers that Heal: How to Use Flower Essences*. Dublin: Gill & Macmillan, 1998.

Kindred, Glennie. *Sacred Celebrations: A Sourcebook*. Glastonbury: Gothic Image Publications, 2001.

Kindred, Glennie, and Lu Garner. *Creating Ceremony*. Wirksworth, U.K.: Glennie Kindred, 2002.

Kollerstrom, Nick. *Gardening and Planting by the Moon 2014*. Slough, U.K.: W. Foulsham & Co. Ltd., 2013.

Lane, Nick. *Power, Sex, Suicide: Mitochondria and the Meaning of Life*. Oxford, U.K.: Oxford University Press, 2005.

Lavender, Susan, and Anna Franklin. *Herb Craft: A Guide to the Shamanic and Ritual Use of Herbs*. Taunton, U.K.: Capall Bann Publishing, 1995.

Linn, Denise. *Sacred Space: Clearing and Enhancing the Energy of your Home*. New York: Ballantine, 1995.

Lonegren, Sig. *Labyrinths: Ancient Myths & Modern Uses*. New York: Sterling, 2001.

Mabey, Richard. *Flora Britannica Book of Wild Herbs*. London: Chatto & Windus, 1998.

MacCoitir, Niall. *Irish Trees: Myths, Legends, and Folklore*. Cork, U.K.: Collins Press, 2003.

McIntyre, Anne. *The Complete Floral Healer*. London: Gaia Books, 1996.

Meehan, Cary. *The Traveller's Guide to Sacred Ireland.* Glastonbury: Gothic Image Publications, 2002.

Melchizedek, Drunlavo. *The Ancient Secret of the Flower of Life.* 2 vols. Flagstaff, Ariz.: Light Technology Publishing, 1999.

Montgomery, Pam. *Plant Spirit Healing: A Guide to Working with Plant Consciousness.* Rochester, Vt.: Bear & Company, 2008.

Nahmad, Claire. *Earth Magic: A Wisewoman's Guide to Herbal, Astrological, and Other Folk Wisdom.* London: Rider, 1993.

Paterson, Jacqueline Memory. *Tree Wisdom: The Definitive Guidebook to the Myth, Folklore, and Healing Power of Trees.* London: Thorsons, 1996.

Rael, Joseph. *Sound: Native Teachings and Visonary Art of Joseph Rael.* San Francisco: Council Oak Books, 2009.

Sands, Helen Raphael. *Labyrinth: Pathway to Meditation and Healing.* London: Gaia Books, 2000.

Scott, Timothy Lee. *Invasive Plant Medicine.* Rochester, Vt.: Healing Arts Press, 2010.

Small-Wright, Machaelle. *Perelandra Garden Workbook: A Complete Guide to Gardening with Nature Intelligences.* Warrenton, Va.: Perelandra, 1993.

Soper, John. *Bio-Dynamic Gardening.* London: Souvenir Press, 1996.

Storm, Hyemeyohsts. *Lightningbolt.* New York: Ballantine, 1994.

Strehlow, Wighard, and Gottfried Hertzka. *Hildegard of Bingen's Medicine.* Rochester, Vt.: Bear & Company, 1988.

Weeks, Nora, and Victor Bullen. *The Bach Flower Remedies: Illustrations and Preparations.* Essex, U.K.: C. W. Daniel Company Ltd., 1990.

Williams, John, ed. *The Physicians of Myddfai.* Facsimile ed. Burnham-on-Sea, Somerset, Wales: Llanerch Press, 1993. (Orig. pub. 1861.)

Woodward, Marcus, ed. *Gerard's Herbal.* London: Studio Editions, 1994.

# Index

Page numbers in *italic* refer to illustrations.

poetry, 41

poisonous plants, 39

pool of reflection, 106–7

Popp, Fritz, 185–86

pork, 55–56

potassium, 242–43

power, 140–41, 153–54

praise, 41

pregnancy, 53

preparation for dieting, 42–44

   Angelica, 220–21

   Blackthorn, 147

   Dandelion, 245–46

   Dog Rose, 103–4

   Elder, 170

   Oak, 126–27

   Primrose, 82–83

   St. John's Wort, 198

Primrose, *pl.4*, 13–19, *13*, 22, 71–92

   description, 74–76

   dreaming, 83–92

   folklore and history, 76–78

   introduction, 71–73, *72*

   modern herbal medicine, 78–79

   plant dieting, 79–83

*Primula vulgaris. See* Primrose

protection, 141, 162–63, 215–16

*Prunus spinosa. See* Blackthorn

purification, 43–44, 45–46

quinessences, 81

radiance, 85

radiation damage, 100

Rael, Joseph, 33–34

Raphael, 221

Raynaud's disease, 217

Red Clover, 166, 242

relationships with plants, 56–57

reproductive system, 99–100

respect, 28

restricted diets, 44

rheumatism, 167

ribbons, 73

roots, 59

*Rosa Canina. See* Dog Rose

sacred fires, 73

sacred objects, 46

sacred space, 45–47

Sage, 45, 193

Sal (participant), 222, 262

salt, 43

Samhain, 69, *158*, 160–61, 283–84.

   *See also* Elder

Saturn, 137

sciatica, 167

Scott, Timothy Lee, 188–89

Sean (participant), 110

Seasonal Affective Disorder, 195

seed plants, 25

self-acceptance, 109–10

self-concept, 226–27, 265–67

sex, 43

sexual energy, 173

shadow self, 48, 140–41

Shakespeare, William, 76

shamans and shamanism, 8, 119

Shekinah, 11–12

shillelagh, 142

showering, 46–47

*Silene stenophylla*, 26

Triple Moon Goddess, 163
Tungus tribe, 8

unity consciousness, 25, 97
upper worlds, 222–23
Uriel, 221
urinary tract, 242–43

Venus, 71, 93, 97–98
vibration, 109–10
vinegars, 60–61, 62
visionary experiences, 254–56
vitality, 141
vitamins, 99, 242

Walters, Merri, 26–27
watches, 47
Water, 49–52
water decoctions, 61
water infusions, 61
Weeks, Nora, 65

West, 50
wheat, 43–44
Wheel of the Year, 68–70, *69*
Wheels of Light, 287
whiskey, 41
Wiccans, 48
Wilson, Tom, 11
wines, 62, 123
Winter Solstice, 143, *182*, 184, 186–87, 284. *See also* St. John's Wort
Wise Women, 8
witches, 141–42
wood, 123
World Tree, *120*
wound healing, 78
wristwatches, 47

Yarrow, 217
Yukari (participant), 203, 252, 253

Zeus, 118

# BOOKS OF RELATED INTEREST

**Plant Intelligence and the Imaginal Realm**
Beyond the Doors of Perception into the Dreaming of Earth
*by Stephen Harrod Buhner*

**The Secret Teachings of Plants**
The Intelligence of the Heart in the Direct Perception of Nature
*by Stephen Harrod Buhner*

**Plant Spirit Healing**
A Guide to Working with Plant Consciousness
*by Pam Montgomery*
*Foreword by Stephen Harrod Buhner*

**The Healing Intelligence of Essential Oils**
The Science of Advanced Aromatherapy
*by Kurt Schnaubelt, Ph.D.*

**Advanced Aromatherapy**
The Science of Essential Oil Therapy
*by Kurt Schnaubelt, Ph.D.*

**Vibrational Medicine**
The #1 Handbook of Subtle-Energy Therapies
*by Richard Gerber, M.D.*

**Dental Herbalism**
Natural Therapies for the Mouth
*by Leslie M. Alexander, Ph.D., RH(AHG), and*
*Linda A. Straub-Bruce, BS Ed, RDH*

**Himalayan Salt Crystal Lamps**
For Healing, Harmony, and Purification
*by Clémence Lefèvre*

INNER TRADITIONS • BEAR & COMPANY
P.O. Box 388
Rochester, VT 05767
1-800-246-8648
www.InnerTraditions.com

Or contact your local bookseller